PSYCHOTHERAPY WITH COUPLES

PSYCHOTHERAPY WITH COUPLES

Theory and Practice at the Tavistock Institute of Marital Studies

edited by

Stanley Ruszczynski

Foreword by

David E. Scharff

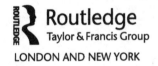

Routledge
Taylor & Francis Group

LONDON AND NEW YORK

Chapter 3: lines from "Here on the cropped grass of the narrow ridge I stand" (1933) by W.H. Auden; from *The English Auden: Poems, Essays and Dramatic Writings 1927–1939*, edited by Edward Mendelson. Reprinted by permission of Faber and Faber. Also from *Collected Poems* by W.H. Auden. Copyright 1937 and renewed 1965 by W.H. Auden. Reprinted by permission of Random House, Inc.

Chapter 9: lines from *Cat's Eye* by Margaret Attwood, copyright 1988 O.W. Toad Limited; used by permission of the Canadian publishers, McClelland and Steward, Toronto, and by permission of Bantam-Doubleday-Dell Publishing Group, Inc.

Chapter 9: lines from *A Passage to India* by E.M. Forster. Used by permission of Kings College, Cambridge, and the Society of Authors as the literary representatives of the E.M. Forster Estate.

Chapter 9: lines from *The Road to Lichfield* by Penelope Lively, published by William Heinemann. Used by permission of Reed Book Services and by permission of Grove Press, Inc.

Chapter 9: lines from *Porky* by Deborah Moggach. Published by Jonathan Cape. Used by permission of Random Century Group and by permission of Curtis Brown Group Limited. Copyright Deborah Moggach 1983.

First published 1993 by Karnac Books Ltd.

Published 2018 by Routledge
2 Park Square, Milton Park, Abingdon, Oxon OX14 4RN
711 Third Avenue, New York, NY 10017, USA

Routledge is an imprint of the Taylor & Francis Group, an informa business

Copyright © 1993 by the Tavistock Institute of Medical Psychology

British Library Cataloguing in Publication Data
Psychotherapy with Couples: Theory and
Practice at the Tavistock Institute of
Marital Studies
  I. Ruszczynski, Stanley P.
  616.89

ISBN: 9781855750456 (pbk)

ACKNOWLEDGEMENTS

I would like to express my thanks to Robert Young, editor and publisher of Free Association Books, for his kind permission to republish Enid Balint's article "Unconscious Communications Between Husband and Wife", which he is to include amongst the collected papers of Enid Balint (*Before I Was I: Psychoanalysis and the Imagination*, edited by Juliet Mitchell and Michael Parsons, Free Association Books, 1993). I am also grateful to Tavistock Publications for their kind permission to republish Alison Lyons' article, "Therapeutic Interventions in Relation to the Institution of Marriage", which had previously been published in *Support, Innovation and Autonomy: Tavistock Clinic Golden Jubilee Papers* (1973), edited by Dr Robert Gosling, for whose generous permission I am also grateful.

I am indebted to Margaret Wilkinson, friend and colleague of the late Alison Lyons, who gave me access to all her unpublished papers, amongst which I found Alison Lyons' article, "Husbands and Wives: The Mysterious Choice". Sincere thanks are due to Evelyn Cleavely and Janet Mattinson, who made time in their busy post-retirement schedules to revise their papers which had previously been presented as lectures. I also give thanks to my current colleagues, Warren Colman and James Fisher, who very generously revised lectures, in the former case, and completed a previously unfinished paper, in the latter, in response to my request to them to do so. Further thanks is also due to Warren Colman for his assistance in checking the references relating to the writings of Jung and his followers; and also for reading and commenting on the Intro- ductory comments preceding parts two, three, and four of this book. Affectionate thanks are due to Douglas Woodhouse, past Chairman of the TIMS. His knowledge of the history, tradition, and philosophy of the Institute was carefully and generously shared with me in relation to chapter one and was much appre- ciated. Isabel Menzies Lyth offered some detailed historical comments, for which I am also very grateful.

More broadly, I am grateful to all the writers, and the whole TIMS staff group, who have waited patiently whilst I have laboured towards the completion of this book. Much thanks is due to Claire Davis, who patiently and skilfully typed vari- ous drafts and revisions of the contents of this book into the word processor. Particular gratitude and affection are due to Margaret Spooner, TIMS Administrator, whose increasingly vocal support and encouragement has been of enormous help.

Finally, both personally and on behalf of TIMS, I would like to express my sincere gratitude to Cesare Sacerdoti of Karnac Books, whose early interest and encouragement, subsequent advice and suggestions, and, more recently, generous patience, has made this volume possible. The highly skilled and efficient editing by Klara King made the final stages of the preparation of this book much less arduous than they might otherwise have been.

CONTENTS

CONTRIBUTORS

All the contributors are past or present senior members of staff of the Tavistock Institute of Marital Studies (TIMS) and have participated in the clinical, teaching, and research activities of the Institute.

Enid Balint   Founder member of the TIMS in 1948 (at which time it was called the Family Discussion Bureau). Staff member and Consultant to present. Training Analyst, British Psychoanalytical Society.

Evelyn Cleavely   Staff member from 1974 to 1989, having taken early retirement. Associate member of staff from 1989 to present. Organizational Consultant.

Warren Colman   Staff member from 1982 to present. Associate Professional Member, Society of Analytical Psychology.

James Fisher   Staff member from 1989 to present. Associate Member, British Association of Psychotherapists.

Alison Lyons Staff member from 1953 to 1977. Consultant from 1977 until her death in 1986. Past Training Analyst, Society of Analytical Psychology and British Association of Psychotherapists.

Janet Mattinson Staff member from 1969 to 1987. Chairman from 1980 to 1987. Consultant from 1987 to present. Professional Member, Society of Analytical Psychology.

Stanley Ruszczynski Staff member from 1979 to present. Deputy Chairman from 1987 (re-titled Deputy Director in 1992) to present. Member, British Association of Psychotherapists.

David E. Scharff

The Tavistock Institute of Marital Studies has a claim to being the most important institution in the world for the psychoanalytic study of marriage. It was, in 1948, the first institution founded along psychoanalytic lines to be dedicated to the study and improvement of marriage, at a time when the stability of marriage had begun to decline around the world. Most early psychoanalytic theorists had been wary of dealing with marriage. Freud assumed that the health and the well-being of the individual were naturally above that of the survival or intrinsic value of relationships. While he understood that children benefited vastly from supportive and loving parents and were lucky indeed if they had parents who loved each other emotionally and sexually, his clinical writing is pervaded with the assumption that family members constitute a frequent and important source of harassment to the psychoanalyst getting on with the job of freeing the neurotic individual from the shackles of his past and of those family members who, in his view, so often offered formidable resistance to change.

It is a curious quirk of historical blindness that Freud could have been so insightful about the value of parental support to young children and yet been oblivious to the similar value to the adult of warm and loving relationships, or, to state the negative case, that he could not see how often adults were devastated by the absence of people who offered effective emotional support, even if such a lack of support occurred largely through the agency of the patient's own self-defeating and relationship-defeating patterns. We owe so much of what we know of individual development to the choices and assumptions that Freud made that we should not be ungrateful, even while noticing, that these same assumptions made it initially more difficult to trace the path of the intrinsic role of, the shortcomings and pathology of, and the ways of offering help to human relationships which we can now see offer a natural complement to the clinical and theoretical findings of psychoanalysis.

It fell to the psychoanalytic study of marriage to begin to redress Freud's original oversight. There were a few early attempts to study marriage, most notably by Flügel in his 1921 book, *The Psychoanalytic Study of the Family*. In his description the family come across as a series of dyads, each negotiating the forces of infantile sexuality and oedipal striving. Although Flügel was restricted by the limitations of his theory and the early psychoanalytic context in which he wrote. he could nevertheless make important observations that presaged the more sophisticated understanding that later theoretical advances in psychoanalysis and family systems made possible, as when he wrote, "in adopting his attitude towards members of his family circle, a child is at the same time determining to a large extent some of the principal aspects of his relations to his fellow men in general" (p. 4). It is of considerable interest to us to note that he expressed regret that so little was known about marital relationships that he preferred to omit discussion of them rather than do them injustice.

The founding in 1948 of what came to be known as the Tavistock Institute of Marital Studies (TIMS), under the leadership of Enid Balint (then Enid Eichholz), began the path of setting this right. Drawing on the advancing edge of psychoanalytic understanding provided by Melanie Klein's description of the infant's use of the mother as an internal object and of projective identification, and in a theoretical climate increasingly supported by an understanding of object relations from the writings of Winnicott, Balint, Sutherland (and through him of Fairbairn), and, later, of Bowlby and Bion, the group made marriage and the marital relationship its focus of study, clinical intervention, and research. The early publications of the group were influential within the sector of the community concerned with the application of psychoanalysis beyond the individual, and especially within the social work community which had a long-standing interest in marriage. Bannister et al.'s (1955) *Social Casework in Marital Problems* was followed by Pincus et al.'s *Marriage: Studies in Emotional Growth* in 1960, and Bannister and Pincus's *Shared Phantasy in Marital Problems* in 1965. Internationally, the word was spread by the publication of Main's "Mutual Projection in a Marriage", in the journal *Comprehensive Psychiatry* in 1966, and most emphatically by Dicks' book *Marital Tensions*, published in 1967. These works demonstrated that an in-depth understanding of marriage offered a great deal to those who wished to improve the health and potential of individuals. Marriage could no longer be considered as a potential hindrance to real progress, but could take its place as a proper focus of study in its own right, as a context for living that reflected the pooled potential of the two partners—a natural setting for growth and development, offering new opportunity while at the same time faithfully reflecting shared difficulty. Through the work of clinicians, writers, and researchers who clustered around the TIMS, clinical work with troubled marriages formed a natural laboratory for the understanding of mutual projective and introjective identification, of adult development, and, as an important by-product, of the family. Clinical sophistication grew. The staff worked at first only with two parallel individual therapies, which were joined at the top by supervision and collaboration. This model was excellent for the initial research into the goodness-of-fit between two individuals. It then led to the model of conjoint co-therapy, which added direct experience about the couple's interaction to the field of observation and intervention. Later, as they studied countertransference and its effect on therapists, the staff offered the option of providing a single therapist to a couple.

The TIMS is no longer alone in its pioneering interest in the application of psychoanalysis to the study and improvement of marriage and the family. In Europe and in North and South America many groups have followed suit, often without awareness of the debt they owe to the TIMS. This collection of essays accomplishes three important tasks of interest to psychodynamic therapists who work with marriage and couples:

(1) It gives a substantive history of the growth of ideas among TIMS collaborators who originally developed analytic approaches to couples and marriage following the founding in 1948 of the "Family Discussion Bureau" by Enid Balint and her colleagues. The early chapters of this book sketch the history of the TIMS through a presentation of the central concepts, giving the reader at the same time a working sense of history and a growing appreciation of clinical application.

(2) Its overlapping montage of contributors and contributions offers several avenues into modern concepts of the work. Thus the concepts of projective and introjective identification, the way that spouses re-find lost parts of themselves in each other, the opportunities for growth and development for the individual in the context of marriage, and the concepts of container/contained—which are understood differently by W. R. Bion and C. G. Jung—are presented from the unique perspectives of the several thoughtful writers.

(3) It offers a new and creative integration of contributions from a Jungian background to marital work. The Jungian contributions complement and amplify the better-known Kleinian, Winnicottian, and Freudian perspectives. By offering this additional perspective, this volume accomplishes a new integration, a step that we grow to see has been missing until now.

The scope of this collection of essays is impressive. It surveys the unconscious underpinnings of the couple relationship, the tension between marital and individual development, and therapeutic approaches to couples. It is perhaps the exploration of the tension between marital and individual development that offers us the most important new material, adding a much-needed corrective to that original assumption of Freud's that they were antithetical to each other. Through the contributions of this book, we begin to see precisely how the well-being of the two individuals is neither simply opposed to that of their marriage, nor is it one-and-the-same thing, but, rather, that individual development and couple relationship are in a dynamic tension with each other. We get a vivid picture of what contributor Warren Colman calls "development in terms of the creative tensions of opposites . . . going on all the time, and . . . moving forward into the future as well as referring back towards the past". Through chapters that reach beyond the tension between individual and couple development to explore the way individuation is made possible or is hampered by marriage, the role of ambivalence in the re-working of the oedipal conflict in couples, and the concept of betrayal of trust in marital breakdown as illustrated in literature, this book also provides a vision of future areas of creative work.

Psychotherapy with Couples is notable for its review of previous contributions of the TIMS, for its balancing of therapeutic and research contributions to the basic psychology of marriage, and for the number of voices from varying but always clear and thoughtful perspectives. Its diversity and its clarity continue the Tavistock tradition, informing the work of students, clinicians, and researchers in the psychology of marriage. Indeed, all practitioners of couple therapy who wish to understand the heart of the psychodynamic contribution and its origins in the seminal contributions of the Tavistock Institute of Marital Studies will find pleasure in this book.

PREFACE

All the chapters gathered together in this volume, except one, were first written as lectures and presented at a variety of conferences and teaching events to a range of audiences with different interests and concerns with the psychological health of the couple relationship. The one exception is the chapter by James Fisher, which the author started to write because of his interest in putting down on paper some of his ideas developed in the course of thinking about and working clinically with couples.

Only two of the chapters have been previously published: Enid Balint's "Unconscious Communications Between Husband and Wife", and Alison Lyons' "Therapeutic Intervention in Relation to the Institution of Marriage". Both are being republished here because they are seminal papers and warrant further exposure to an interested audience.

The chapters have been arranged in an order that gives the collection a coherence. This is always a concern when gathering together a group of papers for publication. Inevitably, there is some overlap and repetition in the content of the chapters, but the editing has been carried out with a view to keeping this to a minimum. The different authors may of course have different views on some of the theoretical and clinical issues addressed, and this variety of perspectives adds to the richness of the volume. The Tavistock Institute of Marital Studies has always taken some pride in maintaining itself as an institution that manages, more or less, to hold the tension between differences. This seems particularly appropriate for a centre concerned with the understanding of and working with the tensions that are inevitable in any couple relationship.

All the staff of the TIMS are trained to work as marital psy-chotherapists, as well as to teach and undertake research. Some have also trained to work as individual psychoanalytical psychotherapists or psychoanalysts. It is interesting to note that amongst those trained for individual work there are Freud-ians and Jungians, with the Freudians spreading across the schools of that tradition locating themselves mostly in the Brit-ish object relations and the Kleinian orientations. What holds the group together—whether trained for individual practice or not, their orientation Jungian or Freudian—is the primary in-terest in interactive process, in intrapsychic and interpersonal object relations, which manifest themselves most powerfully and intimately in the nature of the couple relationship.

The couple relationship, however, is also, to some degree, influenced by external social, cultural, economic, and political factors, which interact with internal, often unconscious, mean-ings and motivations and so create the complex matrix of any long-term intimate couple relationship (see, for example, the TIMS studies of the interaction between work, unemployment, and the couple relationship—Daniell, 1985; Mattinson, 1988; Ruszczynski, 1991). The research activities of the Institute are pursued with this interconnectedness in mind (see chapter one).

Part one of the text offers an introduction to the institution of the TIMS with particular reference to its clinical and teaching practice and its research activities. It is important to give this contextual background, from which the theory and practice described in the subsequent chapters have emerged. TIMS holds the view that clinical, teaching, and research activities are mutually informative and necessarily form the matrix of any centre of advanced study and practice.

Part two concerns itself with the core understanding of the psychoanalytic perspective on the couple relationship—that is, that whatever conscious and considered reasons bring a couple together, hold them together, and sometimes render them asunder, there are also very powerful unconscious meanings and motivations in the partners' original choice of one another and in their subsequent interaction with each other. This fundamental understanding of the couple relationship has to inform whatever therapeutic interventions may be offered to couples seeking help (as well as be taken account of in matters of social policy that relate to couple and family life).

Part three addresses the inevitable, and necessary, tension inherent in any long-term intimate couple relationship—that is, the tension between, on the one hand, the needs of each of the individuals and, on the other, the needs of the partnership aspired to. This tension and its management are at the centre of any personal relationship. It will be particularly powerful in the couple relationship as it is likely to be seen by the couple as a central aspect of their lives.

Part four considers specifically the therapeutic intervention offered to couples and focuses on some of the central clinical issues that are likely to arise in psychotherapy with couples. The conceptual underpinning of the theoretical and clinical work of TIMS is psychoanalytic—with an adaptation of that framework to an understanding of the interaction between a couple and between a couple and the therapist or therapists.

Parts two, three, and four each begin with a brief editorial comment introducing the reader to the chapters contained in that part of the book.

* * *

All the names and details of couples described in the book, for the purpose of clinical illustration, have been altered so as to ensure confidentiality.

THE INSTITUTIONAL CONTEXT

There is no such thing, outside the realms of imagination, as a marriage free from conflict. Such a relationship is not in the nature of human beings. In the depths of our minds we never, throughout our lives, succeed in freeing ourselves fully from the hates and resentments that first arose in infancy. . . . These emotional forces are part of the essential dynamics of our personalities, and they operate intensely in marriage. . . .

Geoffrey Thompson

CHAPTER ONE

The theory and practice of the Tavistock Institute of Marital Studies

Stanley Ruszczynski

I n this introductory chapter I outline the development of the thinking and practice of the Tavistock Institute of Marital Studies as it has developed since its establishment in 1948. It is, of course, not possible in one chapter to trace the entire organizational, intellectual, and clinical life of an Institute spreading over 45 years. I will therefore limit myself to a sketch of the theory and practice of working with couples as it has emerged in the Institute's research, publications, and clinical work. Those who may want to have an overview of the Institute's organizational development can refer to Bannister et al. (1955), Woodhouse (1990), and, more briefly, Dicks (1970).

The Family Discussion Bureau

The Tavistock Institute of Marital Studies (TIMS) came into being after World War Two as a result of the growing political concern for the state of marriage and the family. It is somewhat sobering to read that the particular areas of concern were "in-

3

crease in divorce, separation, marital disharmony, and family tensions" (Astbury, 1955). A contemporary list would, with the addition of child abuse, read rather similarly.

In 1947, against the background of this concern, the Family Welfare Association (FWA), a family casework agency originally established in 1869, initiated what was to become a seminal project. Some of the staff of the FWA were becoming increasingly aware that requests for material help frequently exposed needs of a more personal and emotional kind. The Association therefore decided to offer specific technical help to some of its practitioners in developing their skills to deal with these specific difficulties, focussing in particular on problems of marital relationships (Menzies, 1949). Enid Eichholz (who became Enid Balint in 1953), a senior member of the staff of the FWA, approached the Tavistock Institute of Human Relations (TIHR) for consultative help and advice. TIHR allocated Isabel Menzies (now Menzies Lyth) and Dr A. T. M. Wilson, together with Elizabeth Bott (now Spillius) to work with the FWA on their experimental project (Menzies, 1949; Menzies Lyth, personal communication 1992). This collaboration led to the formation, in 1948, of the Family Discussion Bureau (Bott, 1957). Initially, the group planned to use the title "Marriage Welfare", but decided that this might be seen to be associated with social failure. The hope was that the name eventually chosen—the Family Discussion Bureau (FDB)—could be seen to apply equally to preventative and therapeutic work, and to emphasize the joint client–worker nature of the task (Bannister et al., 1955).

In the Tavistock family: psychoanalytic roots

With the establishment of the FDB and the beginning of the new focus on marital relationships, the caseworkers felt that they needed a deeper understanding of emotional forces and the functioning of relationships to enable them to understand the underlying factors in a marriage. Help, too, was needed to develop the degree of awareness of their own and their clients' reactions to each other, so as to enable them to use the therapeutic relationship as a means of help. Psychoanalysis was seen to offer a substantial theory of relationships, and also a therapeutic goal for effective help. The therapeutic goal was seen to be a need to increase the clients' insight into the unconscious motives that influence the nature of their personal relationships.

Soon after the setting up the FDB, therefore, Isabel Menzies Lyth agreed to explore the possibility of recruiting a psychoanalyst to the group. She approached Dr Michael Balint, who expressed great enthusiasm for the project and became its first psychoanalytic consultant (Menzies Lyth, personal communication 1992). This subsequently developed into a more formal connection with the Tavistock Clinic, and Dr Balint was followed in 1953 by Dr J. D. (Jock) Sutherland and Dr Geoffrey Thompson. Taken together, the psychoanalytic and socio-dynamic orientations of the Tavistock Clinic and of the Tavistock Institute of Human Relations proved to be of enormous value to the FDB, in relation to both staff training and organizational development.

Although the FDB did not formally join the Tavistock Institute of Human Relations until 1956, and then transferred in 1979 to the Tavistock Institute of Medical Psychology (the original body that had set up the Tavistock Clinic in 1920), it has been from its very beginning part of the "Tavistock family" and shared the Tavistock philosophy of applying psychoanalytic principles in its theoretical and clinical approach. In 1968 the FDB changed its name to the Institute of Marital Studies and in 1988 formally appended the name of the Tavistock, to become the Tavistock Institute of Marital Studies. Throughout the history of TIMS, some members of staff, as well as being trained to work with couples, have also undertaken individual psychoanalytic or psychotherapeutic training, at the Institute of Psychoanalysis, the Society of Analytical Psychology, the British Association of Psychotherapists, and the Lincoln Centre and Institute for Psychotherapy. This additional training has never been a requirement nor an expectation, but it has further underpinned the conceptual base of the Institute, which has always been "catholic" in its theoretical and technical development. It has been influenced by Jungian thinking, by the work of the British object relations school (especially Balint, Sutherland, and Winnicott), and by the work of Klein and Bion.

The interrelated functions

When the FDB was established in 1948 it defined its tasks as threefold:

> To provide a service for people seeking help with marriage problems; to devise techniques appropriate to such a service, and evolve a method of training caseworkers; and, to find out something about problems of inter-personal relationships as they reveal themselves in marital difficulties. [Astbury, 1955]

This stemmed directly from the Tavistock focus, which had been, since its establishment, that of understanding and treatment, research, prevention, and teaching to specialists and non-specialists (Dicks, 1970).

The present-day TIMS retains precisely these same aspirations and has the same functions as in its beginnings: psychotherapy with couples, training and consultation, and research and clinical studies. These tasks are, of course, interrelated and each informs the others in a mutually nourishing interaction. The many publications that have emerged from the Institute have recently been critically appraised in an essay–review (Haldane, 1991).

To outline the theory and practice of the TIMS would require a constant interweaving between the three functions: clinical observation may lead to a research project; the research produces new concepts and frames of reference, which may be written up in papers and books; publication of these may lead to training and teaching events; teaching may inform supervisory and clinical practice, and so on. Within the psychoanalytic tradition there has always been interconnectedness between theory and clinical practice. As Kurt Lewin asserted, "there is nothing so practical as a good theory" (quoted in Woodhouse, 1990). The historical picture I give, therefore, tends to be more disjointed than the reality of the interconnectedness between the three functions. The chapters that follow and make up this book then discuss in greater detail some of the clinical thinking and practice of couple psychotherapy at the TIMS.

Theoretical underpinnings

In the first two publications to emerge from the TIMS (Bannister et al., 1955; Pincus, 1960), the two sets of authors outline the psychoanalytic view of human growth and development that shapes the internal world of the child and continues to influence adult relationships.

> The dynamic theory of behaviour offered by psychoanalysts seemed especially appropriate for marital problems. In recognizing the importance of unconscious forces in mental life, it gave a basis for understanding and dealing with the irrational and emotional elements in personality which often prove so intractable in family tangles. [Bannister et al., 1955]

In the course of infancy and childhood, the developing human being builds up an unconscious inner world made up of the images corresponding with the earliest experiences of significant others and how these satisfied or frustrated his needs and wishes. Because the infant's emotional and intellectual capacity is very limited, he is unable to apprehend the "reality" of those around him and tends to experience emotions in extreme form. "Good" experiences become idealized and raise the phantasy of omnipotence, and "bad" experiences become terrifying and persecutory. This inner world has a compelling reality, and external situations are interpreted in accordance with it. The ways in which the human being relates to his environment and to others in it are characterized by his earliest experiences. In the course of normal growth, the testing out of phantasies against normally favourable reality slowly bridges the gap between the two, and a more realistically ambivalent sense of internal and external relations emerges. However, residues of the more primitive images remain and may be reactivated by certain situations, relationships, or life events. Each new relationship throughout life is experienced against the background of these internal images, the more "mature" as well as the more primitive.

This concept of personality offers a framework for understanding the unconscious meaning of many of the disharmonies of an individual's relationships. It also offers a framework within which to understand the way a couple relates to the psychotherapist. "Transference attitudes can often be observed and used even without detailed factual knowledge which would enable the (psychotherapist) to 'account for' them" (Bannister et al., 1955). The recognition by the psychotherapist of these repeated unconscious patterns of relating is as important as a precise and detailed knowledge of the facts of the couple's relationship and of each partner's life. "The history of the patient's object relations comes alive in the transference" (Joseph, 1988).

Choice of partner

As well as offering a way of thinking about the nature of couple interaction, and how this will be re-enacted in the transference relationship to the psychotherapist, psychoanalytic theory also suggests ways of understanding partner choice.

Partner choice always involves conscious and unconscious parts of the personality. The strongest bond between a couple may well be the harmony of their unconscious images and patterns of relationships. "Sometimes the partner may seem to characterize a repressed or split off part of the other's personality; often very dissimilar partners seem to find in each other what they have most sternly repressed in themselves" (Bannister et al., 1955).

By mutually receiving one another's unconscious projections, each partner gives the other an initial feeling of acceptance and attachment. This externalization of the internal conflict into someone who has to be contended with each day may enable that part of the personality to become gradually more tolerable within the self; however, it may alternatively produce a fierce effort to control or punish it in the partner. Tensions within a couple relationship can therefore be thought of as internal conflicts externalized and acted out in the partnership. In this sense the couple relationship can be thought of as a mutual transference relationship.

Shared phantasies and shared defences

These processes of projection and projective identification (as well as the resulting introjection and introjective identification) are part of normal average human development, and continue to be employed in all relationships. The mutual acceptance of the other's projections constitutes the unconscious attachment that the couple will have to each other and will consist of shared internal phantasies and shared defences. If too much of the personality is projected or if too little is found to be acceptable and so slowly taken back, these mechanisms can impoverish the personality, which has in effect disowned parts of itself. It will also result in weak boundaries—the sense of self and sense of other is confused by the projective system. If this defensive posture is held too rigidly, the partners' shared phantasies and illusions and their shared defences will become defining and restricting characteristics of their relationship.

This, then, becomes the focus for the couple psychotherapist's therapeutic intervention. In this sense the patient for the couple psychotherapist is the couple's relationship—the interaction between the two partners—rather than either or both of the individuals. The dynamic nature of the interaction is, as it were, between the two partners' split-off and projected parts of themselves, as located in the other, the force with which these are projected, and how they are recovered and dealt with by the other. At the extreme, each partner is in effect not relating to a separate other but to the disowned self, projected into and identified with in the other. The exploration of shared phantasies in couple psychotherapy may allow the projected attributes to be found less terrifying and eventually felt to be capable of being taken back. The psychological boundaries between the two partners become more clearly established, and so internal and external object relationships are subsequently modified.

* * *

Alongside the development in the 1960s of the theory of couple interaction and its implications for couple psychotherapy, the TIMS was also teaching what it was learning itself to various other practitioners from many disciplines who may in the course of their own professional practice deal with couples and families and who will therefore benefit from an understanding of couple interaction.

Much of this teaching was conducted in groups, which became "training laboratories": the Institute staff would test out their theories and develop methods of application for those practitioners in other agencies and institutions.

> It is no accident that practitioners concerned with marital work, and therefore with manifestations of intrapsychic processes in inter-personal relationships, should find themselves paying attention to the group as a vehicle for containing and working-through the emotional impact of learning and working in this field. They could not be unaware, in themselves as in their clients, of resistance to personal change. . . . Bion (1961) observed and documented processes by which members of a group can unconsciously co-operate in avoiding the struggle with its real task. The parallel with ways in which couples can unconsciously co-operate to maintain illusions about themselves and each other is striking. [Woodhouse, 1990]

One of the most important developments in the work of the TIMS emerged out of a series of teaching seminars run for social work supervisors in South-West England between 1965 and 1974.

The reflection process

Following Heimann's seminal paper on countertransference (Heimann, 1950), in which she argued that the psychotherapist's feelings towards the patient need to be conceptually separated from the psychotherapist's transference to him, the hypothesis was offered that the psychotherapist's feelings and attitude to his patient may be understood as *more* than simply his personal reaction, his transference, to the patient. A growing interest therefore developed in the use the psychotherapist may be able to make of his affective responses. This development challenged the idea of the psychotherapist's "neutral" stance and obliged a review of Freud's perhaps confusing suggestion that psychotherapeutic treatment "may be compared with a surgical operation" (Freud, 1916–17). In simple terms, it is hardly possible to be working with a patient without, to some degree, consciously and unconsciously, becoming involved in the relationship and therefore affected by the patient.

Heimann initiated the process whereby psychotherapists began to think more about the nature of their emotional involvement with and response to their patients. Rather than seeing it simply as a personal response that had to be avoided, it began to be recognized as something necessarily being unconsciously stirred up by the patient and therefore needing to be understood. "The issue is not between detachment and involvement, but between objectivity in the presence of involvement" (Dicks, 1967). This theoretical and clinical development was substantially aided by Klein's discovery of schizoid defence mechanisms, particularly projective identification (Klein, 1946), which was subsequently developed, primarily by Bion (1952, 1955), to be understood not only as a mechanism of defence, but also as an unconscious means of communication from the patient. Countertransference, the feelings and reactions stirred up in the psychotherapist, came to be seen as a major source of information and therefore a psychotherapeutic tool, though it remains a controversial and much discussed issue in psychoanalysis.

The basic understanding is that some of the feelings stirred up in the psychotherapist have been projected into him by the patient, both for defensive, evacuative purposes but also as a means of unconsciously communicating certain aspects of his internal world. The task for the psychotherapist is to become consciously aware of what is being stirred up in him, make some sense of it, and offer some understanding to the patient through an interpretation or comment. It also came to be understood that if this initially unconscious communication cannot be translated into the psychotherapist's consciousness, for whatever reasons, then that which has been stirred up in him may be reflected, or acted out, either with the patient or in other situations—for example, in a supervision session or case conference, or in relation to other colleagues.

This thesis was developed in an interesting way by Searles, who suggests that the emotional experience of the supervisor in relation to his supervisee may have significant informational value about the relationship between the supervisee and the patient being discussed. He suggests that "the processes at work currently in the relationship between patient and therapist are often reflected in the relationship between therapist and supervisor" (Searles, 1955). He calls this "the reflection process". Unconsciously the supervisee, unable to process and free himself from the patient's projection, may find himself re-enacting in the supervisory setting something of what has been projected into him by the patient (Mattinson, 1975). The supervisor, at one remove from the powerful unconscious defensive processes of the therapeutic encounter, may be freer to make sense of and understand some of the unconscious messages being reproduced in the supervision.

In case discussion groups this same phenomenon also occurs and may even become exaggerated. The behaviour of the discussion group may offer some indications of what has not yet been made conscious and understood in the psychotherapeutic relationship being discussed (for a vivid illustration of this, see Joseph, 1985, pp. 157–158). Within the TIMS, the clinical case conference, in fact, played a key role in the development of its practice of couple psychotherapy. This was particularly so in relation to the growing understanding of transference and countertransference phenomena, as revealed in the co-therapists' working relationship during the course of the presentation of their therapeutic work to the clinical case conference.

This reflection process works in two ways—from the therapeutic work to the supervision, and from the supervision back to the therapy. The psychotherapist is the linking common factor. The process is, of course, easier to describe than to observe and make use of. The more powerful and subtle the projection, the less likely it is that the supervisor or the group will be able to interpret it. But, as with countertransference, of which it is an enactment, great care needs to be taken that what is being re-enacted in the supervision or group discussion is actually to do with the patient. Supporting evidence from history, for example, is useful corroborative information.

A further dimension of this reflection process is that, as said earlier, it may also be enacted between colleagues. It becomes very clear therefore that when, for example, two co-therapists are offered to a couple being seen in psychotherapy, some of the difficulties experienced by the patient couple may become reflected in the working relationship between the two co-therapists. In this, what might be called, marital countertransference (Ruszczynski, 1992), the co-therapist couple may need to make sense of something between themselves—put there unconsciously by the patient couple through projective identification—before the patient couple are able to do likewise. The co-therapist marital countertransference work, if successfully achieved, may produce a verbal interpretation, or, at times, the co-therapists' struggle to make sense of their anomalous interaction may be unconsciously communicated to the patient couple, who are then enabled to attempt their own understanding. It has been argued, for example, in individual psychoanalytic work, that toleration of the countertransference by the psychotherapist can, for some patients, be mutative in its own right (Carpy, 1989).

This reflection process between the two co-therapists, the marital countertransference, is one very important clinical rationale for giving couples two psychotherapists. It is particularly valuable if the predominant defences include splitting, as the two psychotherapists may find that between them they hold the full picture of the couple's shared internal world, either split between the two partners of the relationship or split between them as a couple and an external object (Ruszczynski, 1992).

Summarizing briefly from a historical point of view: the development of a psychoanalytic understanding of couple interaction in the 1950s (Bannister et al., 1955; Pincus, 1960) led to developments during the 1960s and 1970s in the clinical technique for couple psychotherapy, and the teaching of this to other practitioners (Bannister & Pincus, 1965; Guthrie & Mattinson, 1971; Institute of Marital Studies, 1962; Mainprice, 1974; Mattinson, 1970, 1975). During the latter part of this time it began to be clear that the process of interaction being studied between partners, between co-therapists, between therapists and supervisors could also be usefully and constructively applied more broadly. Obholzer has summarized this view recently by stating that there is

> no conceptual difference or clash between our approach in understanding an individual, a couple, a family, a group or an institution. The difference rests solely upon where one draws the boundary of one's field of observation and intervention . . . the unconscious processes in all these settings have identical origins. The basic underlying principle is that institutions (and here I am referring to the individual psyche, the marital psyche, the group psyche and the institutional psyche) defend themselves against the anxiety and pain inherent in the workings of the system by a variety of defences, mechanisms and techniques. [Obholzer, 1987]

Working intensively with couples in psychoanalytic couple psychotherapy offers a unique opportunity to study processes of human interaction at great depth—processes that operate less obviously in all relationships, be they personal, social, professional, or organizational.

Out of the consulting room: action research

As a result, the TIMS began to broaden its research interests away from the clinical research of the consulting room activity into the world outside. To some degree this had already been initiated. Research previously carried out by a new member of staff was published: it showed that individuals who had previously been resident in a hospital for the mentally handicapped managed noticeably better as couples than they had as individuals (Mattinson, 1970); and a consultative input to a children's hospital attempted to develop an approach to helping sick children, through working with the marital interaction of their parents (Mainprice, 1974).

A new strand began to develop in the work of TIMS as it attempted to examine, via collaborative action research projects, the relationship between the personal lives of couples and aspects of their external environment. Teaming up with various welfare agencies, TIMS staff would personally participate in the work of an agency, or offer workshops to the agencies' practitioners, or often both, to learn at first hand, through participatory experience, about the area being researched.

A non-specialist setting

The first of these major research projects was with an inner-London Social Services Department. For three years, four TIMS staff members worked alongside basic-grade social workers, offering to work with couple problems as they presented themselves to a non-specialist agency, looking to learn from the setting but also to contribute from their specialist knowledge (Mattinson & Sinclair, 1979). Very few couples were referred to the department, and even fewer were referred specifically for problems in the couple relationship. However, it became clear that accommodation, financial, psychiatric, and child-care referrals were often symptomatic of severe conflicts between couples. (It is interesting to note that it was exactly this same experience that some Family Welfare Association caseworkers had had in the 1940s, reinforced by the views of some Citizens Advice Bureaux staff, which led to the setting up of the specialist Family Discussion Bureau, whose concern it was to try to understand and tackle the underlying problems located in the couple's relationship).

To carry out the therapeutic work required of them by these often very demanding clients, the TIMS staff used not only their familiar theories of marital interaction and the reflection process, but also Bowlby's theories on attachment and loss (Bowlby, 1969, 1973a, 1980) and the theory of institutional defence (Jacques, 1955; Menzies, 1970). The rather depressing outcome was to suggest that these were often the most needy and disturbing clients, but that local authority departments were not necessarily structured in a way that might best support the practitioners who were working with them.

The first baby

The next major research project was an exploration of the impact on the couple of having a first child. The idea for this originated from clinical experience of couple psychotherapy, which suggested that the psychological adjustment from a twosome to a threesome presented some couples with substantial psychological stress and disruption. Working collaboratively with health visitors and the parents themselves, the TIMS staff examined the emotional adjustments required of the couple and how they attempted to prepare themselves for the arrival of the baby. One of the most interesting findings to emerge from this research suggests that "the personal meaning and implications of parenthood could not be learned in advance but had to be discovered through experience" (Clulow, 1982).

The children of divorce

One of the areas of public and political concern in Britain for some decades now has been the growing divorce rate. Statistical evidence suggests that well over one-third of first marriages and approximately half of second marriages are likely to end in divorce. Whatever the legitimacy might be for a couple to end their partnership, the impact of such an event on the children of that relationship is substantial. TIMS members of staff undertook research into those situations where the divorce court became involved in child-care arrangements subsequent to a divorce because the divorcing couple themselves were unable to come to a mutually acceptable arrangement. The research findings suggest that unresolved attachments to the now divorced partner, and all the other historical and contemporary losses that this process might activate or reactivate, are often played out in relation to the making of decisions about what is in the child's best interests (Clulow & Vincent, 1987).

Work and loss of work

Another major social phenomenon of the 1980s was unemployment—an issue revisiting Britain again in the early 1990s. As a result, again of clinical experience, where a growing number of couples approaching the TIMS for couple psychotherapy were presenting themselves after one or both partners had been made unemployed, the Institute set up a research project to examine the psychological impact of loss of work on the couple relationship (Mattinson, 1988; Ruszczynski, 1991). It became very clear that to understand the psychological meaning of unemployment, the psychological meaning of work had to be better understood first (Daniell, 1985). This parallels the now understood need for a divorcing couple to make conscious and to give up that which may have been invested in their marriage, now lost, before they are able to manage their separation reasonably amicably.

What emerged from the research into the psychology of unemployment was that, to some degree, particular jobs are chosen, or transformed, so as to meet unconscious internal needs and conflicts. Once secured, this allows other areas of that individual's life to be free from the pressure to deal with these psychological requisites. When the job is lost, therefore, the loss includes that which had been taking care of these emotional requirements. It is likely, in such circumstances, that the couple relationship may be turned to to meet some of these needs and may well not be able to do so. One of the most important outcomes from this research was that for those people who are psychologically dependent on their work activity to secure their identity, the loss of that work may lead to a major crisis in their sense of personal and interpersonal self.

Telephone helplines

Child sexual abuse is the other current social issue that demands attention and understanding. The TIMS work in this
area was of a different type in that it arose as a result of a
request for a training programme from volunteers involved in
the running of a telephone helpline for parents who feared that
they might abuse their children. This project did not include a
direct interest in the couple relationship—by definition, it was
not available for scrutiny. As already outlined above, however,
an understanding of processes of interaction learned about
from the study of couples is applicable to other processes of
interaction, including the one here between the telephoning
client and the helper on the other end of the telephone line. The
write-up of this research (Colman, 1989) includes a discussion
of the very difficult borderland between reality and fantasy,
particularly in relation to sexuality and sexual abuse.

Collaboration and anxiety

The findings from the most recently completed research programme have now been published. "Collaboration involves the
exploration of differences and the revelation of uncertainty",
writes Woodhouse (1990) with reference to this publication on
the dynamics of institutional collaboration (Woodhouse &
Pengelly, 1991). All the above areas of research, briefly mentioned, have involved collaborative processes between the TIMS
staff and the other agency, between the agency and its own
staff, between the staff and the clients, and, if the clients are
couples, between the couples themselves. This most recent research was exactly about anxieties inherent in any collaborative enterprise and how these can undermine attempts at
co-operation. It is perhaps particularly fitting for the TIMS staff
to undertake such a research programme because by
Woodhouse's definition of collaboration, quoted above, as involving "the exploration of differences and the revelation of uncertainty", marriage and the couple relationship must rank as
an exercise in collaboration par excellence.

* * *

During the 1970s and 1980s, whilst much of this research was taking place, the TIMS continued to develop its clinical expertise and to offer teaching and consultation. The Institute produced another text on couple psychotherapy (Clulow, 1985) and a book for the layperson (Clulow & Mattinson, 1989), and it celebrated its fortieth anniversary and published the papers given at the celebratory event (Clulow, 1990).

The three functions today

The TIMS continues to pursue its three interrelated functions, sometimes struggling to do so against financial and other pressures. The pursuit of any one or pair of activities may lead to the exclusion or attenuation of the other or others, and if the work to maintain the at times uneasy equilibrium between the three is given up, the Institute may cease to be technically viable and is likely to atrophy as a centre of advanced learning and practice.

The TIMS has an extensive teaching, training, and consultation programme, ranging from the intensive in-house specialist diploma in marital psychotherapy to a very broad range of courses, workshops, seminars, and consultation programmes for social workers, probation officers, psychologists, medical personnel, clergy, lawyers, psychotherapists, and counsellors, as well as their supervisors, trainers, and managers. The TIMS trains specialists to work with couples, but the substantial part of its teaching activity is to other professional practitioners, whose pursuit of their primary task may be enhanced by knowledge of processes of interaction and collaboration.

Research work at present is concentrated on three areas, all in their very early stages. One is a project monitoring the Institute's own clinical practice, which may result in a second phase of the research into actually evaluating marital psychotherapy, and the delineation of a typology of marital problems. The second research programme relates to couples who are undergoing hospital treatment for infertility. The focus of this project is on the couple relationship at a time of major stress and into the counselling requirements that would best meet the needs of such couples. The third area of research interest relates to an access centre that is used by children and parents following the breakdown of the couple relationship.

Whether any of these preliminary programmes will develop into major pieces of research will emerge with time. All, of course, are important and potentially instructive for all practitioners working in the areas of couple and family life.

Clinical work

Underpinning, informing, and sometimes stimulating its research and training activities is the clinical work of the TIMS. Through the couple psychotherapy undertaken within the Institute, clinical skills are continually challenged and refined, and limitations in theory and technique are brought to light for further development.

As psychoanalytic understanding has deepened and explored yet earlier processes of interaction, so it has aided attempts to deepen understanding of the nature of the couple relationship. The many and complex fears and phantasies, joys and pleasures of earliest object relationships will be reactivated in the interaction between partners, as well as in their joint relationship to the environment they live in, perhaps the most important being their children if they have any. The deeper the theoretical understanding, the more likely that the subsequent clinical technique that emerges will increase therapeutic effectiveness.

When the TIMS first started to work with couples in the late 1940s and 1950s, its model of working was with the two partners of the couple relationship each having their own psychotherapist and each partner–psychotherapist pair *meeting separately*. No doubt this was to do, in part, with the model of individual psychoanalysis. It may also have been to do with the, at the time, underdeveloped understanding of the theoretical and technical dynamics relevant to psychotherapeutic work with couples. The concept of projective identification, amongst others, became very important in the advance of the theoretical

understanding of unconscious partner choice, unconscious collusion between a couple, and shared anxieties and defences.
This theoretical advance also aided the technical understanding
and use of transference and countertransference phenomena.

During the 1960s, couples began more often to be seen
jointly, together with the two couple psychotherapists (see, for
example, Bannister & Pincus, 1965). By the 1970s working
with couples included the possibility of working either all together as a foursome, or in parallel single sessions, or a combination of the two, the choice of model at any particular time in
the course of the therapy being diagnostically indicated partly
in relation to the nature and degree of splitting and projection
evident in the couple's interaction (Lyons, chapter ten, this
volume). In simple terms, the thinking is that if the couple use
excessive splitting and projection, as well as blame, denial, and
the other more primitive defences, then they need to be seen
together, so that the two sides of the split can be located in one
room and for the two psychotherapists to be witness and
party to the nature and degree of the splitting and projective
processes. Further, with the development of the concepts of
countertransference and the reflection process, the foursome
setting was also seen to offer the opportunity for the co-therapist pair to be a therapeutically useful arena, both for the projections emanating from the couple and for the processing and
understanding of the purpose and meaning of the use of this
mechanism.

If a couple are not using such primitive defences but have a
greater degree of psychological maturity and some capacity for
ambivalence and concern for the other, then the work can proceed in either foursome sessions or in parallel single sessions.
In either setting, with less splitting and blame taking place,
both partners will be able to acknowledge their part in the
tensions of their relationship, and so the couple psychotherapy
is able to proceed.

Individual sessions, running in parallel for the two partners,
may be required if the internal object relations of each partner
in the couple are highly persecutory and if paranoid anxieties
predominate—the couple may not be able to be in a room together and be able to share the two psychotherapists. In such a
diagnostic category individual sessions might establish some

basic trust and benevolent transference, leading to the possibility of foursome couple work, which could then be implemented.
Individual sessions are also indicated with partners who may be
developing more depressive and less persecutory object relations, as the one-to-one sessions offer more direct and detailed
psychotherapeutic attention to the painful transition that this
psychological development requires.

By the 1970s and through to the clinical practice of today,
TIMS couple psychotherapy may be in the foursome setting.
This is the product of a continuing development of theories of
marital interaction as an application and adaptation of psychoanalytic concepts. It relates to an increasingly sophisticated
understanding and use of the concepts of projective identification, particularly as enacted in the transference and countertransference, both between the couple and between the couple
and the psychotherapists. It also relates to an increasing clarity
that it is the marriage, or relationship, that is being attended to.
In some cases individual sessions, in parallel, continue to be
the appropriate model of therapeutic intervention. This will be
made available according to the needs of the couple, and its
possible or actual use symbolizes the tension inherent in any
and every couple relationship—that between the individuality of
the individuals and the partnership they aspire to. In other
cases a single therapist will see the couple. Whether particular
couples are better aided therapeutically by being seen by one
therapist or by two co-therapists is, alongside the issue of the
gender of the therapist(s) (Morgan, 1992), among the current
clinical research interests of the Institute.

A CONCLUDING COMMENT

The study of the couple relationship may offer psychoanalytic
theory an opportunity to explore what Winnicott refers to as
"the third area". This third area he defines as that of cultural
experience, which he sees as being a derivative of play. The
other two areas are that of inner psychic reality and the actual
external world in which the person lives (Winnicott, 1967).

I would like to suggest that this "third area" may equally well be thought of as being that of the *relationship* created by the couple's interaction with each other. The couple relationship exists in the space between the two partners to the relationship.

The couple relationship is par excellence the arena for the constant interplay between the intrapsychic and the interpersonal. It is pivotal between inner psychic reality (including the perception of the other) and external reality as represented by the otherness of the other. The couple relationship may sometimes actually produce a third—a child—as a true product of the interaction between the two. This creative outcome depends on the fruitful intercourse between differences.

The theory and practice of the TIMS has always been a rich and complex but mutually beneficial interweaving of the different strands of the Institute's activities: clinical practice, teaching, and research (clinical research and external action research). This interweaving seems particularly appropriate to a unit whose primary focus of interest is the interaction of a couple in a relationship.

The chapters that follow describe a psychoanalytic understanding of the nature of couple interaction and the subsequent clinical practice appropriate to couple psychotherapy.

PART TWO

THE UNCONSCIOUS CONTRACT IN THE COUPLE RELATIONSHIP

> Experience drives one relentlessly to the conclusion that beyond what is consciously known about by the partners concerning their choice of each other, each, at a deeper level, recognizes aspects of themselves, of which they are not consciously or willingly aware, in the person of the other.
>
> *Douglas Woodhouse*

INTRODUCTION

The focus of theoretical and clinical interest for the couple psychotherapist is the interaction between the couple—the relationship mutually created between the partners. The nature of this relationship, changing over time and particularly affected by the events of the natural life cycle, is the product of the externalization of internal images and object relations shared by the partners. Unconscious partner choice is made on the basis of the other's receptivity to projected aspects of the self. This process of mutual projective identification is the central mechanism in the establishment of a couple relationship—the unconscious attachment will be due in part to the mutual acceptance of the other's projections.

The four chapters that follow discuss this unconscious arrangement in the couple relationship from slightly different theoretical perspectives. All agree, however, that the intimate couple relationship offers the possibility for the working through of unresolved internal conflicts and anxieties.

In "Unconscious Communications Between Husband and Wife" (chapter two), Enid Balint reminds us of Freud's discovery of the transference relationship that develops in the two-person relationship of psychotherapist and patient. In this relationship, impulses and phantasies from the past are transferred into the present relationship. This is not unique to the analytic relationship and arises spontaneously in all human interaction. Enid Balint suggests, therefore, that Freud would have been aware that this same reawakening of earlier inner impulses and anxieties would emerge in the intimacy of the couple relationship. (An important difference, of course, is that the task of the psychotherapist is to make these transference feelings conscious; a couple are not likely to be consciously aware of what is brought into their relationship in this way.)

Enid Balint argues that the couple relationship is a particularly receptive forum within which internal needs and anxieties are likely to be expressed and seek some response or even resolution. Her chapter describes the various ways in which a couple unconsciously communicate and express their respective impulses and anxieties to each other, and how this communication shapes the nature and development of their relationship.

Alison Lyons' chapter, "Husbands and Wives: The Mysterious Choice" (chapter three), takes up the same theme, but from a Jungian perspective. She suggests that the choice of partner is substantially determined by the drive to individuation, which "leads people to choose partners who will activate undeveloped aspects of their own selves" (p. 48 below). This is not to say, however, that people only form relationships with opposites. It is necessary, she says, for some degree of similarity and identification to exist if the conflicts and anxieties inherent in the individuation process are to be felt to be manageable.

Both Enid Balint and Alison Lyons also refer to the conflict and pain inherent in psychological development and growth and emphasize that this is an inevitable aspect of any healthy couple relationship. This is the theme of Evelyn Cleavely's chapter, "Relationships: Interaction, Defences, and Transformation" (chapter four). She writes that such conflict can only be healthily managed in a couple relationship if the partners have first established a trustworthy defensive system. In this way every couple relationship has to manage a necessary and inevitable tension between the more developmental and the more defensive aspects of their interaction.

Warren Colman's chapter, "Marriage as a Psychological Container" (chapter five), gathers in many of the ideas touched on in the other chapters. He draws on Bion's concept of "container–contained" and Winnicott's concept of "holding" to inform his discussion of the capacity of the

couple relationship to function as a forum for psychological development. This is, of course, inherent in the intimacy and intensity of a committed couple relationship.
When this ordinary everyday therapeutic capapability of
intimate relating breaks down, the aim of couple psychotherapy is to offer the couple an opportunity to reflect
upon themselves and their interaction so as to consider
whether it may be possible to restore and enhance the
capacity of the relationship to function again as a psychological crucible for integration.

The concept of the unconscious contract in the couple
relationship, therefore, offers a way of understanding the
nature of partner choice and couple interaction and delin-
eates the task for the couple psychotherapist when a couple present themselves for help.

CHAPTER TWO

Unconscious communications between husband and wife

Enid Balint

One of the cardinal problems that interested Freud right from the start of his work was how to understand the individual's difficulties in terms of his early history within the family. This means that right from the beginning psychoanalysis recognized that the atmosphere of the family, which is created primarily by the interaction or collaboration between two partners—husband and wife—and is later complicated by the arrival of the children, was of paramount importance for the future development—which more or less means adaptability—of any individual. In spite of this, there has been remarkably little research, and little has been written by psychoanalysts on the dynamics of these marital interactions. There have been some exceptions, mainly in the 1920s (Groddeck, Deutsch, and Horney, for instance, had some important contributions to make on this topic), and during the past 15 years or more [the author wrote this in 1968 and so is referring to writings from the early 1950s onwards], in this country and in America, a few psychoanalysts have turned their attention to the study of marital interactions and have used insights that they had gained as analysts to help them to understand and to attempt to formulate theories about family behaviour.

In my work at the Tavistock Centre with the Family Discussion Bureau we have, right from the beginning of our work, in 1948, tried to understand marital difficulties by focusing our attention on the interaction between the two partners. That is to say, we have studied the marriage as an entity rather than two people as separate and isolated individuals. [When this chapter was written, the Tavistock Institute of Marital Studies was operating under its original name—the Family Discussion Bureau; see chapter one.]

Perhaps marriage somehow goes beyond the natural field of interest of psychoanalysts whose main field of interest is the individual alone—his urges and drives and his relation to his own private life, which includes his dreams and fantasies, his hopes, disappointments, and wishes, about his family as he first knew (or imagined he knew) them. Whereas, in addition to the individual's internal life of hopes, disappointments, fears, and wishes, his partner's internal life and how these two affect each other, interact, or do not interact with each other must be considered if theories of marital interaction are to be formulated. Furthermore, even these interactions cannot be examined in isolation, because the comparative simplicity of the marital relationship is made even more complex when each child is born, not only because of the introduction of a new individual with his own strivings and his own personality into the home, but also because of the changes in the parents brought about by each pregnancy.

The basic atmosphere, though, in a marriage that is created by the interaction between the husband and the wife will not, probably, be fundamentally changed, and my presentation would become too complicated if I were to include the effect of the children on it. So, for the purpose of this chapter, I will discuss marriage as if it consisted of two people only, but I will not be forgetting the relevance of the presence of children in a family and the changes brought about by each one.

Our concern, therefore, will be to study how one person's individual life and expectations and hopes and fears dovetail into and influence another's. We must not forget, however, that this interaction is also studied by sociologists, anthropologists, and social psychologists, partly on the basis of what a third and uninvolved person can observe. They discuss their findings, using concepts like interpersonal relationships, family process, family interaction, and others. They attempt, for instance, to find satisfactory ways of describing the kind of family that produces or contains a schizophrenic or a delinquent child.

Freud, and after him all psychoanalysts, while paying little attention to marital or family interaction, noted and studied in detail the importance of one particular kind of two-person relationship: that which exists between a patient and his analyst. He found, for instance, that if a patient's expectations and, can one say, illusions about his analyst are not understood, the analytic treatment does not proceed. He also found that all patients have unrealistic ideas about their analysts. As early as 1895, he called this kind of relationship "transference" because it "stemmed from the impulses and fantasies which were aroused and made conscious during the progress of analysis— when the person of the physician replaces an earlier person" (Freud, 1895d). (That is to say, feelings are transferred from that earlier person onto the analyst.) After a time he noted also that transference does not only arise in psychoanalysis but that it arises spontaneously in all human relationships. The difference, he says, is that it is revealed in analysis, whereas in other human relationships we are largely unaware of its manifestation. So, Freud, although never stating it explicitly, must have been well aware that impulses and fantasies that stem from the past are reawakened in marriage too, and that husbands and wives must have unrealistic ideas and expectations about each other in marriage. The difference is that it is hardly ever recognized between the husband and wife as it is between the patient and his analyst. But clearly it must be of the greatest importance to them and to the family atmosphere that is created by them.

Freud realized that an individual cannot be studied on his own; that is to say, his conflicts and difficulties in relation to another person have to be taken into account, as well as his wish to modify his behaviour to suit the other person and his wish to modify his partner to suit him. An individual, in fact, is never in a vacuum. In spite of that, the analyst is concerned with the experiences of one person only. In order to explain these experiences Freud developed a two-prong theory.

(1) The theory of instincts: in this theory instincts are understood as dynamic forces that are on the borderline between biology and psychology. They create urges or drives that force the individual to pursue certain goals; for instance, his sexual drive forces him to seek a partner, his hunger drive forces him to seek food, and so on.

(2) The second theory is more complicated. It is based on history and accident. Here, once again, there are forces in the individual, but these originate from accidents in the special history of that individual, and they can be seen to create tendencies or drives in him to repeat what has gone before. For example, he may find himself repeating certain forms of behaviour and find himself unable to accept other forms, however gratifying they might be. He may have a tendency towards reparative acts, towards feelings of resentment, or towards desires for revenge, and so on. This theory can be called the "developmental theory".

The two theories, that of instinct and that of development, both have characteristic forces. Both of these theories are needed to explain the internal experiences of one person and are both also needed if we are to understand interpersonal relationships.

But things become even more complicated when we intend to study the ways in which two people communicate. Perhaps, in fact, this is a further reason why marital interactions have not been studied by analysts. It is difficult enough to understand the varied and contradictory forces, and the fantasies by which they become conscious, that are awakened and transferred in the comparatively simple analytic situation, where only one person's feelings, ideas, and fantasies are verbalized and where only one person transfers (because the analyst has learnt in his training to understand and control his own transference when treating patients). So perhaps the cross and contradictory transferences in marriage are felt to be too complicated to disentangle and so have been left on one side. But if we are to discuss communication in marriage, we must see how much of this kind of interaction can be clarified by psychoanalysts. So let us start by describing some simple and well-known ways in which husbands and wives communicate.

Words form only a small part of communications in general. We communicate also by the way we move, by our facial expressions, by our silences, by the way in which we give things or do not give things to each other, and so on. When I speak about communication in this chapter, I mean communication in this wide sense. In marriage non-verbal communications are particularly important. Often the person who wants to communicate does not himself know consciously what he wants to say—or he may not even know that he wants to say anything at all. Part of our mind is unconscious, and this speaks also. In addition, our partner's conscious mind may not notice that anything has been said when we communicate with him, although his unconscious mind may set in motion a response. Or, to put it another way, a husband may communicate with his wife without being aware that he has. Or the wife may be aware that something has been meant (by, for instance, a gesture or a frown) but may not be quite clear what it was and may not know consciously that she has responded to this. Winnicott writes of a baby only registering, but not hearing, the mother's silent communication (Winnicott, 1968). What I have just said is that this kind of communication is highly important in marriages too, but that, in addition, in marriages it can be seen to be a two-way process. (It probably is also a two-way process between a mother and her baby, but we can only observe it reliably in the mother.)

Husbands and wives fit into each other's needs in the most subtle way, even in the worst marriages, and even, in fact, when there are many areas where they do not fit in at all. For instance, a husband who naturally has a rather small appetite may find himself eating and enjoying huge meals because his wife thinks he likes them. Or a wife who says she is too tired to go out in the evening may unconsciously be doing so because it suits her rather timid and depressed husband.

Let us look at some marriages in greater detail. For instance, in one case a husband came home from work, and his wife told him that she had had a terrible day with the children but everything was all right now and that supper was ready. In saying this, she unconsciously said to her husband that she had had a horrible time and would perhaps like to have a drink, or be kissed and made much of. The husband failed to note the communication and instead found himself going into the garage to see whether the car was all right. He was unaware that he was responding to his wife's unconscious communication, and she was unaware that his withdrawal to the garage was a result of it. Married couples act constantly on one another in this way; they modify each other's behaviour in the most complex manner, and they rely upon each other to do this. This is a part of their daily lives—the atmosphere in the family; the whole feeling of family life would be unthinkable without it.

To an outside, uninvolved person, what appears to be an antagonistic communication can easily be a loving one. That is why it is so difficult for an uninvolved observer to understand what his observations (which can be absolutely accurate) mean to the two partners in a marriage.

When people live together in the same setting over a period of time, they are aware that they are in communication and may value each other's presence when nothing at all seems to be going on between them. For instance, they may not be able to get down to some quite simple job unless they are both in the house together. Each one knows that his activities are enriched by the presence of the other, although neither might become aware of it except in the other's absence. This kind of thing is usually meant when people talk about "home". Most people know that they like to be at home, that they may like or dislike getting home after a holiday, and they may not even be aware that they are not really at home when the other one is away. Even if a married couple are on bad terms with one another and feel hostile and irritated about something, they still (and it may be particularly then) may want the other to be there so that they can carry on with their lives in an ordinary way. In addition to its obvious connection with childhood, there are various theoretical ways of explaining this state of affairs.

For instance, we talk about one person putting part of himself into another person and then feeling lost without that part of himself, but unconsciously recognizing it and feeling whole again when relating to it in the other person. This kind of process happens automatically. We are certainly not aware that we do it. We sometimes get rid of parts of ourselves we do not like in this way and blame our partners for having them. Or we may feel empty of our loving feelings, which we are only in contact with when our partner is there. Or we could say that we need our partner to see that we are loving, to confirm our loving feelings, in order to take them back into ourselves and feel good again.

No two homes have an identical atmosphere, no two couples communicate in the same way, but in each there are some characteristics on which that particular marriage is based. These characteristics may not be noticed by either partner as they are there continually and are created by the two of them together, by their two individualities, personalities, and transferences—conscious and unconscious. Here are some examples.

The dynamic structure of one marriage was that the wife had to appear weak and in need of protection. But she had to be just weak up to a point. It was not tolerable for either of them if she was too weak. The wife was happy when she was made to feel rather weak up to that point and if at these times she enjoyed it when her man was strong, there was harmony between them. If the mutual expectations were apart, then there was that much tension between the two. Things could never be absolutely right, for both of them, all the time. Marriages are often, as was this one, a mixture of satisfaction and tension. There is often a subtle balance between the two.

Another example: in one marriage the wife appeared to run and control everything. Observers from the outside were rather sorry for the husband, and the husband sometimes complained about his wife's bossy manner. But, up to a point in this marriage, the wife's bossiness suited both partners, and when the point was roughly the same for both of them all went well, but if not then there was trouble.

One husband and wife always appeared to be very loving and considerate with each other when they were together. The wife seemed most grateful for her husband's help and care—particularly when she had her frequent, but short, bouts of depression. To an outside observer they suited each other very well; and so they did, but not in the way that showed itself. The wife, in fact, was very frightened of possible outbursts of temper, and her husband prevented these by his kindness. But, by so doing, he prevented her using herself and overcoming her fears of what her temper might do. This suited her husband, because he also was frightened of violence. Their compulsory love-making consisted mostly of petting; penetration was too frightening for both of them. This suggested that the couple could not be violent sexually either and that was perhaps one of the reasons why they could not achieve a family. The unconscious communication from the wife to the husband was, "look after me please, save me from my awful violence". His answer was, "yes, I will". So he agreed with her that she needed to be saved from her violence, and this suited him very well too, even though he had to live with a sense of resentment without knowing why.

Another rather similar couple found a different solution. In this marriage the wife appeared to be a timid person who kept herself to herself in her home and made very few demands upon her apparently cheerful, strong, virile husband. The husband was very much admired at parties, and his wide circle of friends pitied him for having such a quiet, retiring, and unamusing wife. They all thought he was marvellous to put up with her so loyally. In reality, though, the situation was very different. The husband was a frightened man and not very potent. He needed to be admired, but he kept people at a distance because unconsciously he always feared he would be found out. His wife fitted in with him because she needed to be on her own a good deal and did not like to be interfered with. She wanted to go her own way and encouraged her husband to be sociable. In fact, she was a rather aggressive and tense woman who sometimes exploded and wanted a good row with her husband—partly so that they could get close afterwards and become intimate with one another. But she knew in some way that she had to act with great care and caution, because if the row became too heated, the husband would feel really threatened and unable to enjoy the kissing or lovemaking afterwards. Their private hidden satisfactions were not apparent, but both husband and wife were careful to keep their public image alive, not only because, in a vague way, they knew that by so doing they were protecting each other, but also because they were only dimly aware of the true state of affairs.

In many marriages there is a basic communication that things should be as they are, but if things become too tense, there is, as a rule, little possibility of a discussion about them because neither partner is consciously aware of his expectations and wishes. Neither of them knows or is conscious of what they communicate, by their actions or by the atmosphere that they create, so that they cannot put things right by words when their actions breakdown. Degrees of consciousness can vary. Some people are sometimes fully conscious of what to expect from their partner and themselves. Some may not want to admit what they know. Some may be willing to accept it if it is forced upon them, and so on. These kinds of atmosphere characterize a marriage and are kept alive constantly by apparently trivial and everyday kinds of communication. In the marriage I referred to earlier, where the wife complained about the children, the wife's basic expectation was that she should be rather over-pressed and martyred, that she should communicate this to her husband in a roundabout way, and that he should sometimes accept it and do something for her and sometimes reject it and get out of her way. The basic expectation for both of them was that the wife should not say, "I'm tired, please give me a drink", but that she should formulate her request and her complaint indirectly. Trivial communications sometimes have far-reaching implications. They can convey hostility or love. But they may not be verbalized, nor may they, without grave disruption, go beyond the boundaries that are silently and unconsciously agreed upon between the two of them.

We often find that it is just as difficult for people to express openly that they love and appreciate one another as it is for them to be critical. Many people, in fact, are less inhibited when they are critical than when they are affectionate and appreciative. Sometimes, if they do try to express their feelings, they may find that what they say is inadequate; it is too little or too much; or it is inappropriate.

If we want to understand these apparent contradictions, we must bear in mind that what people feel is only partly conditioned by the present. Everything we say or do is partly influenced by what has happened to us in the past; sometimes events are too closely connected with the past, and they cannot be spoken about in a satisfactory way.

There are ways of overcoming these difficulties. For instance, husbands and wives give each other pet names, which,

when used, express much more than could be expressed otherwise and produce a particular atmosphere. They remind the
couple of intimate occasions from the past. The use of the name
may recreate a whole scene or fantasy from the past or an
event so that here there is no need to talk about it. Even here,
though, it may be that the importance of the remembered or
fantasied event transcends the event itself, and this can be
because the event itself was a repetition or a reminder of some
even earlier event or fantasy, which may have occurred before
the husband and wife knew each other. But in spite of this, it
suits both of them.

I have already said enough to make it clear that there are
many possibilities of misunderstandings as well as under-
standings in marriage, and some conscious and many more
unconscious ways of dealing with them. How, then, do these
habitual forms of communication originate? On what does a
person's ability to communicate depend? We have already seen
that it has something to do with transference, with expectations
and fantasies that stem from the past and impose themselves
on the present. So let us briefly survey our ideas about how
they develop. Before doing so, however, I would like to stress
that whatever tendency in an individual I describe, it is never
the only tendency present at any given moment. There are usually many contradictory ones, and at any given time one of
them may be the strongest, but it may be displaced at the next
moment by another. I am referring here to what Freud called
the principle of over-determination (Freud, 1900a).

In every human relationship primitive elements are always
present. These primitive elements have the structure of an exclusive two-person relationship, and so clearly they are especially important between husbands and wives. We think that
they originate from the earliest experiences in the life of every
individual, when he lived in a primitive world where only he
and one more person—his mother—mattered. These early experiences form the basic structures of our personalities. This
simple exclusive two-person relationship does not last too long,
because we soon become aware of the existence of a third person: of our father, with all the complications and conflicts that
come about in a triangular situation—the oedipal phase, with
which I am sure you are all familiar. For every individual, how-

ever, the situation is soon complicated once again by the emergence of other people, first by members of the family, then by neighbours and friends, and then, finally, by even larger parts of society. The introduction of new people always creates problems and conflicts, which must be solved one way or another, sometimes well, sometimes not so well, and sometimes very badly indeed; and, as I have just said, when talking about over-determination, very often not one but many complications arise at any one time.

The individual's position in his family and later the family's position in society offer or even impose on each of us certain solutions that can be called family traditions, social conventions, customs, and so on. The individual's "vocabulary" of communication depends, then, on his way of integrating all these factors and finding a solution to many contradictory internal wishes and external conditions for himself and for the people he loves.

To sum up, a person's ability to communicate and relate depends firstly on his innate possibilities; these are difficult to isolate but we assume that they are present; secondly, on his early experiences, all of which continually act on him and modify him throughout much of his life. His adaptability is not settled once and for all at the primitive level of his relationships, but changes and improves or deteriorates. Although these processes continue well into adulthood, an individual's adaptability can never be absolute. He will always have some unalterable prohibitions and commands forced upon him by his early attempts to find satisfaction for himself and for the people he loves. His communications are an expression of the pressure caused by these problems.

To return to one of our previous examples, I shall isolate one particular trend in the development of the woman who did not complain in a direct way and had to engage her husband's sympathy indirectly. She was the second child in a large family, and when she was very young she was entrusted with the care of her younger brother. It came to light during her treatment that as a child she could never ask for love directly from her mother or her father but often got herself into trouble so that the mother was forced to leave the other children and look after her. The father was away from home during a good deal of her childhood. All this made the little girl very guilty and anxious. When, because of her own guilt feelings, she made it difficult for her mother to look after her in a satisfactory way, she felt neglected and resentful. All her life she found it difficult to ask for what she wanted, and during her treatment she made it very difficult for the analyst to help her, although she was miserable when she got no help. She talked a lot about the problems of other people in her sessions and found reasons for being late or staying away. In her marriage her husband responded to this kind of behaviour by appearing to ignore it, but it came to light in his treatment that he always wanted to be asked for help, and he became angry and could do nothing unless he was explicitly wanted. He felt, in spite of this, some hostility to demanding women, particularly to those who were nearest to him and whom he loved the most. He had not been able to feel very close to his much-loved mother, who had been a rather depressed woman and who had needed help but who had prevented her son from helping her, even in small ways around the house, because of her depression. So in this marriage neither the husband nor the wife were able to communicate with each other directly, but they were able, in spite of this, to find a way to help each other—true, in a rather indirect and cumbersome way, but in a way that was, nevertheless, available to both of them. This pattern was also a disturbance in their sexual relationship. They enjoyed intercourse, but both prevaricated so much that they seldom had it.

One of the most striking, and perhaps encouraging, things that psychoanalysts have discovered is that people never give up trying to put things right for themselves and for the people they love. Even when they may appear to be doing just the reverse, we often discover that what appears to be the most desperate and useless behaviour can be understood as an attempt to get back to something that was good in the past or to put right something that was unsatisfactory. Over and over again people come back to their failures in an attempt to remedy them, even if they cannot help repeating the same failure over and over again.

We could say, then, that in marriage we unconsciously hope to find a solution to our intimate and primitive problems, particularly to those that we feel we cannot communicate socially in an acceptable way. We are inescapably driven to make relationships in the hope of communicating something that was unacceptable in the past, and we hope to find a person to love in a way that will satisfy ourselves and our partners. Each individual is usually aware of some of his hopes and his needs in relationships, and he may be embarrassed by some of them and unconscious of many. In spite of this, he will still, often unconsciously, hope to find satisfaction for them all in marriage. Unless we are too discouraged, we all continue to expect to have someone with whom a gratifying form of communication can be established. Each person hopes to be accepted by and acceptable to his partner, whatever he is like.

Two people, then, partially aware of what they are seeking and not fully capable of expressing it verbally, do, in the end, find each other and decide to marry. They will find reasons for their choice of partner which are sensible and rational to both of them, but, in addition, they will be unaware of many of the underlying reasons for their choice. If this is true, and so much is inaccessible to rational decision, it seems remarkable that there can be satisfactory marriages. But we know quite well that there are. This should fill us with respect for the unconscious. In this chapter I have tried to discuss some of the forces used by the unconscious to achieve this aim.

In marriage the nature of the relationship is unconsciously agreed upon between the two partners, but it is capable of change for better or for worse as time goes on. No two marital relationships have identical atmospheres, identical characteristics, but in all marriages there are unconscious factors that are important to that particular couple. The individual differences that are present in every marriage are the result of the married pair working out between them a solution that satisfies them both, or one that is the only solution they are capable of at that particular time. And, finally, these solutions are not consciously decided upon. They just seem to happen. They are the result of a multitude of communications that are partly expressed in words, many in acts, but which may also be silent and barely visible.

Marriage is a uniquely difficult relationship, because in it two people voluntarily come together for life and form a relationship in which they hope to satisfy each other in a great

many areas of human functioning, not only in the sexual area
and the parental one, but in many more besides. That this
succeeds as well as it does is, as I have already said, perhaps
one of the surprising things. However much we may complain
about the frequency of marital difficulties and marital break-
downs, I think we ought to credit and be impressed by the fact
that there is so much marital harmony and satisfaction. True,
the harmony and satisfaction are often more difficult for the
outsider to see than the disharmony and dissatisfaction, but if
one takes a closer look they can be found to be present even in
the most unexpected places. We have found, in our therapeutic
work with marriages under tension, that hidden loyalties and
satisfactions are our most valuable allies.

Husbands and wives:
the mysterious choice

Alison Lyons

There is a sizeable amount of literature, mostly sociological but also psychological, about the influences governing marital choice. In particular the psychoanalytic view of the influence of parental images has been thoroughly detailed. It may seem that the element of mystery is, in fact, lacking. It is, after all, common knowledge that men marry their mothers, even if it is less commonly known that women are sometimes likely to do the same. These are well-explored premises. Nevertheless, because of their unconscious nature, these choices still have a mysterious quality that constantly invites further exploration.

There are, it has been said, no truly right or wrong choices. It is only their implementation that may or may not be within an individual's capacity. Any true and lasting bond between two people, married or not, does after all require for its maintenance more than a system of mutual projections. It requires the continuing conscious effort to recognize the reality of each partner by the other as well as the capacity to forgive each other for not turning out to be all that was originally projected. Couples need to be able to accept each other, not only as the people they happen to be, but also as the people they are in the process of becoming. It is a tall order, but it is basically one with which we are all familiar. It involves the attempt to convert what was originally a largely unconscious, instinctive choice into a conscious commitment. The passion that carried the individuals into the relationship has to be converted into the on-going energy that will make it work. The constant effort that this transformation requires, the doubts and fears that accompany it, as well as the exhilaration of discovery that it can afford are not exclusive to personal relationships. They are inseparable from commitments of any kind.

Allenby describes the problem very well (Allenby, 1961). She gives the example of a nun referred to her in middle age, who dreamt repeatedly of a handsome young man approaching her bed. These dreams were experienced by the nun as nightmares, which left her in a state of terror. Her confessor told her that they were temptations of the devil that she must forget and think only about the will of God. This, as Allenby points out, was entirely logical from an orthodox Catholic point of view (at any rate at that time—now, thirty years later, she might have received a more imaginative response). What remains certain is that, if all available libido is turned towards God, backed up by the power of the Church, then rebelling instincts will eventually subside, but the patient will fall ill in some way, cut off, as she will be, from any relationship to her erotic feelings and phantasies. In this instance, Allenby found it impossible to question effectively the authority of the father confessor and so was unable to help her patient to face what had been repressed. She had, in fact, taken her vows very young, when she could not possibly have understood what they implied. "It seemed to me", writes Allenby, "that she was being deprived of the value of realizing consciously what precisely it was she had to give up. Her vows of chastity and obedience had been an unconscious sacrifice of instinct, they lacked the ethical quality of choice" (Allenby, 1961). Perhaps she did need to look back at what she had given up and grieve for it.

When one of the partners in a marriage begins to get restless, the nightmare/dream that leaves him or her in a state of mingled terror and excitement may well be the approach of an actual rather than a dream lover. The same dilemma between inner potential and collective standards then ensues. If the partner yields, without question, to the pressures of society, financial considerations, the needs of the children, and so forth—all very powerful realities—and resolutely dismisses not only the would-be lover, but also the chance to work through the feelings that want to be recognized and valued, believing simply that there is "no choice", then the likelihood is that either another lover will shortly appear, or a period of depression will set in which may, with luck, push the sufferer into some attempt to find out what it is all about—to find out, that is, about the aspects of the self that are asking to be realized but are not in the marriage. In doing this, he will have to become aware of the complexities of intra-psychic and inter-personal conflicts, of the necessity for choice, and also of the process of his own individuation. Without luck, the relationship gets stuck, sours, or becomes just a ritual.

I realize that the example that I have given makes it sound as if I am referring exclusively to marriages in which the partners are trying to adhere to vows originally made in Church, whereas there are, of course, several different sorts of marital partnership currently established between men and women, and for many of them there is no question of a life-long commitment, nor any expectation of sexual fidelity. However, in any partnership that is of more than a temporary and casual nature—"any true and lasting bond"—there will inevitably be a commitment of some kind, and the dynamics of choice will continue to apply.

The poet W. H. Auden has most beautifully described the dilemma I have been struggling to express. He is referring to a special kind of commitment—that of people generally, all of us—to each other in the aftermath of the industrial revolution, and although this was written in 1933, it has a terribly contemporary ring.

> To all logical precision we were the rejoicing heirs.
> But pompous, we assumed their power to be our own,
> Believed machines to be our hearts' spontaneous fruit,
> Taking our premises as shoppers take a tram.
> While the disciplined love which alone could have
>   employed these engines

Seemed far too difficult and dull, and when hatred
  promised
An immediate dividend, all of us hated.
Denying the liberty we knew quite well to be our destiny,
It dogged our steps with its accusing shadow
Until in every landscape we saw murder ambushed.

[Auden, "Here on the cropped grass of the narrow ridge I stand"]

Mary Williams has made a clear statement about the degree of individual development required for the sort of "disciplined love" that is needed for the task of transforming an instinctual into a conscious choice. Answering the question, what is the criterion for a successful mature marriage, she says that it depends on a sufficient degree of ego development having been established before the "fatal compulsion" (which is what Jung calls falling in love). This enables the individual, "to weather disappointments and to work through them towards a more real value judgement of the partner's strengths and weaknesses in relation to those of our self. Only then is a partnership built on mutual co-operation possible" (Williams, 1989). In her paper Mary Williams also gives an account of Jung's ideas about marriage, many of which are contained in his paper, "Marriage as a Psychological Relationship" (Jung, 1925). She refers to Jung's concept of marital choice as part of the individuation process, and she comments that, "The notion of unconscious choice is as old as Plato at least. He had the idea that man and woman were once one, that they got separated and spent their lives trying to find the other half again. Jung's discoveries in this respect were more scientific" (Williams, 1989). They were, in fact, developed from his word association experiments, conducted in the first decade of this century. Mary Williams goes on to show how Jung's concept of individuation and the cluster of theories around it have been developed by psychoanalysts.

In his book, "Jung and the Post-Jungians", Andrew Samuels adds a new group to the various schools of psychotherapy, which he calls the "unknowing Jungians" (Samuels, 1985). By this he means that in psychoanalysis there have been many inaugurators of change and development who reflect, without knowing that they do so, an already established Jungian re-orientation of psychoanalytic theory. Among the developments to which Samuels refers there is one, related to the individuation process, that is of special interest to anyone who is concerned about marriage. This is the concept developed by Erikson and Milner that the search for personal integration and wholeness is a more central issue than is "genitality", or even "sanity". From early in his work, Jung was writing about the urge to develop one's own personality, and in "Psychological Types" he develops this theme, defining it as the process of individuation: a movement towards wholeness by means of an integration of conscious and unconscious parts of the personality (Jung, 1921). There has been in this connection some question about the word "wholeness" that inevitably carries with it the idea of health, whereas Jung's original description suggests that it is a process of becoming oneself—whatever one has it in one to be. In other words, individuation demands a recognition and acceptance of parts of the self that are initially repugnant and may, indeed, be pathological.

Following Jung, my main thesis concerning the choice of marriage partner is that the unconscious drive to individuate leads people to choose partners who will activate undeveloped aspects of their own selves. This may lead, sometimes, to marrying a partner who resembles the parent who originally "had it all". Such an idealized choice offers a path on the one hand to individuation, and on the other to a source of continuing envy. Or, again, they may choose a partner who offers a refuge for their own rejected dependency needs—a partner needed but then despised. To maintain that there is a bias in the choice of partner towards one who carries a rejected or undeveloped aspect of one's self is not the same as to suggest that people tend to marry their opposites. Indeed, there is evidence to show that successful marriages seem to be based on a sufficient but not too great similarity between the partners. As in any other form of partnership, there needs to be a sufficient degree of identification to make conflicts manageable. However, when in marriages conflicts cannot be integrated within oneself but remain outside, as part of the "marital warfare", destruction of the once prized object may occur and divorce ensue. But the partners' search for their still undiscovered selves will continue and can lead them into sequential marriages to partners, all of whom bear an uncanny likeness to one another.

An alternative to the flight into divorce may be that the couple, or one or other of them, seek psychotherapeutic help. Then, in confrontation with the unknown figure of the therapist, the search will continue via the transference. As the patient unconsciously tries to turn the therapist into the partner of his choice, sooner or later the therapist may find himself experiencing reactions very similar to those that are attributed to the spouse. He will then have to ask himself why this transaction has to be repeated, and what might be at stake. Like the nun's recurrent dream, this repeating pattern might be an indication that the patient needs to begin the struggle to withdraw projections and so convert an inter-personal into an intra-psychic conflict. He may now be ready to face the realization that needs can never be wholly met and to digest his own irritation, not to say rage, on discovering that disappointments and even a sense of outrage are an ordinary everyday part of living.

In making an assessment of the patient's readiness for such an undertaking, the therapist has to take into account not only his stage of development, but also the strength of the partner's need to maintain the *status quo*. I examine this in greater detail later. At this point I want to illustrate what I have been saying, but not with a "case"—what follows is taken from a popular magazine (*Options*, February 1985, pp. 86–88). It is the supposedly true story of a couple, who, for the purposes of the article, called themselves Brian and Sarah.

> Brian and Sarah had been married for twelve years, and they had no children. He was a very successful 50-year-old English company director, and she was a 37-year-old American accountant. He described himself as a humdrum, unemotional sort of guy, who had married someone who screams her head off for five minutes and then shuts up because she has got it out of her system. He found this "very refreshing". She described herself as having been a free-wheeler from the age of eighteen, but she had always known that underneath the free-wheeling she hankered for security. She had seen Brian as security incarnate. After six years of marriage, their mutual frustration had come to a head. Sarah became aware of it first. Her secure Brian had turned into a "stick-in-the-mud". She began looking for more excitement. She thought

of divorce. But then she began to realize that being tied to Brian was *not* the chief cause for discontent. She realized that, like many young women, she had settled down before she felt she had fully tested herself in the world at large. In doing so, she now realized, she had taken herself away from the real independence and self-knowledge she had always been seeking, and at the same time she had created for herself an illusion that she was lost in the marriage. She now accepted that the fact of the matter was that she had never "found herself" in the first place. So she felt she needed to go back to the point years ago, when she had broken off that all-important search.

She decided to take a year off and trek round the world on a very limited budget. To her this meant going in search of herself. But most of this, she said, had not been all that clear to her at the time. It was actually Brian who had more of a grasp of what was happening. He encouraged her to act. He said: "The thought of losing her while she was away didn't occur to me at the time, because of my much greater concern, which was that I would lose her if she didn't go." He wanted to offer financial help with her project, but she preferred to rely on very prudent budgeting and her own resources. She knew instinctively that this was something she had to do entirely alone. Both admit to having been very scared. "We didn't talk about the future, because we both recognized that there was a very real possibility that we might lose each other." When they actually said good-bye, both believed, but neither voiced, that it was the end of their marriage. And in a way, it was an end to that marriage, because when they rejoined each other it was in a different relationship.

Sarah's was neither a comfortable nor a conventional tour. She stayed in primitive villages, she back-packed through the Himalayas, and she worked as a Red Cross volunteer. He, on the other hand, did not sit at home moping. He took himself off to parties, had the occasional affair, but came at length, as his wife did, to the conclusion that what he really wanted was to continue being married to his present far-away partner.

All their friends thought she was a monster for leaving him. They felt very sorry for Brian and were convinced that she was out of her mind. Her mother refused to speak to her. However, the couple wrote to each other regularly, and Brian was the only person that Sarah felt had really understood why she was compelled to take such a risk with their relationship. Eventually, when she returned after the year, both felt they had learnt to appreciate each other in a way that would not have been possible if they had not been willing to disturb the *status quo*. Both of them had had the opportunity to view their relationship from a new perspective. *"Being so completely separate* puts things in a different light." "Most important, it made us both aware that we did have a choice." Both realized that they could renew their marital commitment or stay apart, and the knowledge that they had chosen to stay together rather than simply feeling trapped together made all the difference.

The big break, as they called it, had taken place six years before. "The change in Sarah," said Brian, "is enormous. She's not the same person." She agreed. She knew now that the source of her previous malaise had not really been lack of excitement in their relationship, but was the reflection of much deeper problems. She realized that she had once bought wholesale the idea that she had to be "an achiever", that otherwise she would be a failure. Even though she had had a good job and a quite "good-enough" marriage, she lacked the positive self-definition that she had once thought only high-flying success could bring. Distancing herself from Brian and the fulfilment of a dream had helped her to realize the sense of self she had so desperately needed. Back from her trip, she decided to write a guide-book for women travelling alone. It did not sell. Had she been the woman she had been before her travels, she would have been devastated. But now she was not. Writing the book was like the trip—a feat of considerable discipline and courage, qualities that could now be called upon in all areas of her life. Suddenly to achieve something for the sake of proving her worth seemed a childish exercise. She had at last liberated herself from the collective idea of success. She was now doing part-time voluntary work and said she had never felt "more complete". It could be said that she had found the security she once vested in Brian in her own tested ability to surmount difficulties and to survive hardship.

Despite the happy outcome friends and neighbours still felt that her year off had been an act of supreme selfishness. Brian argues that "selfishness implies being spiteful in one's lack of regard for other people's feelings, and I don't think what she did was a matter of disregard for me". Sarah said, "It was selfish, but if the relationship was to survive I really had to do it".

This case is so unusual and yet so usual. If they had had children or less money, this "acting-out" of the search for self would have been an impossibility. Yet how often have all of us heard this story and tried to help couples find a way to that psychic distance so necessary for their growth and so difficult for them to envisage, except in terms of physical separation. It is, after all, as Sarah said, "being so completely separate" that "puts things in a different light".

Fortunately for Brian and Sarah, there was a sufficient degree of ego development and of identification with each other to allow them to forgive each other and thus themselves for their disappointments.

Sometimes, if a couple come into therapy at the point of disillusion, they come believing sincerely in their wish for change and in their mutual need to work towards emotional maturity. They then find, to their surprise, that even so they still unconsciously respond to one another in ways that interfere with each other's development. This husband, who from the beginning had been "the secure one", must have had to exercise great self-discipline to prevent himself from deprecating his wife's attempts in the direction of maturity. The wife must have had to resist the temptation to collude with his fear of her "growing up" and away from him by accepting his financial help for her project. Had she given way to it, she would have put herself under an obligation that she would afterwards have come to resent. She would not then have felt that she was free to choose.

In his writing on individuation Jung never discounted the importance of the cultural environment. Whereas it was a sign of their ego development that Brian and Sarah could withstand the powerfully expressed disapproval of their relatives and friends, one of the most tragic couples that I can remember were not so well equipped.

These two had made what all their friends and neighbours could only regard as a disastrous match, and when the time of disillusionment set in, the wife, feeling herself quite isolated, took her unconscious revenge on everyone by killing herself.

I am about to finish these thoughts about the mystery of who marries whom, and I am wondering why this particular case, striking its bleak note, should have occurred to me at this point. Marriages do not result in suicide very often—or is there a sense in which they do? Do partners more frequently than we would like to recognize give up their struggle to individuate in favour of accommodation to a more comfortable seeming *status quo*, yielding, as Sal Minuchin, the family therapist, has said, to that "miscarriage of intimacy which tends to sacrifice individuation to loyalty" (Minuchin, 1984). Patients, as they begin to make different adjustments and develop different needs, do sometimes have to choose between their marriage and their analysis. Peter Giovacchini, describing this phenomenon, says that in his view—and it is the view of many psychoanalysts—marriage partners choose each other because of an unconscious need of someone with a particular psychopathology. He sees this as a purely defensive measure necessary for ego stability (Giovacchini, 1961). I have been trying to illustrate Jung's additional insight—that is, of the purposive nature of such unconscious choice. Jung has also described the pitfalls and extreme difficulties involved in realizing this purpose. So I will let him have the last word.

A good thing is unfortunately not a good forever, for otherwise there would be nothing better. If better is to come, good must stand aside . . . so that anything destined to be better first appears in evil form. . . . To develop the personality is a gamble, and the tragedy is that the demon of the inner voice is at once our greatest danger and an indispensable help. It is tragic, but logical, for it is the nature of things to be so. . . . Can we therefore blame humanity . . . if they erect protective barriers . . . and point out the roads that wind safely past the abyss? But, in the end . . . everything could be left undisturbed did not the new way demand to be discovered, and did it not visit humanity . . . until it is finally discovered. The undiscovered vein within us is a living part of the psyche . . . a flow of water that moves irresistibly towards its goal. [Jung, 1925]

CHAPTER FOUR

Relationships: interaction, defences, and transformation

Evelyn Cleavely

I n 1960 the Family Discussion Bureau, as the Tavistock Institute of Marital Studies was then known, published a clinical and theoretical book entitled *Marriage: Studies in Emotional Conflict and Growth* (Pincus, 1960). It remains one of the Institute's best-sellers.

The book explores, in relation to the psychodynamics of the marriage relationship, the principle that the tension between opposing or seemingly incompatible forces facilitates opportunity for growth and development. It makes the statement that without conflict there is no growth. Central to understanding this factor, however, lies a paradox: tension arising from conflict provides at the same time equal opportunity for both creative *and* destructive potential. You cannot have one without the other. A quick glimpse at modern history gives evidence to the existence of this paradox. There has never been a century, as far as we know, quite like the one presently drawing to its close, when man has been so inventive and creative. Neither has there been a century like it, which has so demonstrated man's capacity to destroy. So much has been achieved for the enhancement of future generations, but never has mankind been so uncertain of having a future, and never has a century been *so* concerned with conservation and the uncertainty of its own completion. Creativity casts its shadow before it, and the tension between creative and destructive potential is akin to the paradox of life and death itself. One is outraged by death and yet somehow knows that living in its full sense is dependent upon accepting the certainty of one's own dying. There is a quality to life and living made possible only because life as we know it comes to an end.

It is impossible, I find, to think about the marital relationship and about my work with couples without thinking about the meaning and significance of life—its riches, uncertainties and horrors—and the capacity to live it. For the marriage relationship is intrinsically concerned with man's need to regulate the conflict between the two fundamental needs necessary to his growth and development: the need for intimacy and the need for autonomy. The management of the inevitable feelings of love and hate towards the same person, which this conflict arouses, is central to understanding the psychodynamics of the marital relationship.

The study of marriage is rich in content—unique, in fact— because it is the *only* heterosexual relationship between two people of more or less equal maturity where sex is overt. The understanding of the psychodynamics of interactive processes made possible by the study of marriage relationships has wider implications and is applicable to other relationships, to family and organizational networks (see chapter one, this volume). However, within this undoubted truth we discover a further paradox. Resistance towards attempting to make sense of a couple's interaction and distress may often lie within the therapist and belongs to the therapist's own internal world as well as to that of his clients.

Marriage comes close to the bone for all of us, whether or not we are actually married. We all have an image of a marriage within us, an image greatly influenced by the quality and nature of how we experienced and perceived our parents' marital relationship and how these parents negotiated the child's inclusion and exclusion from that relationship. It is often difficult, therefore, to distance our internal worlds from the impact of our clients' marriages. For in coming close to their conflict and pain, we sometimes come uncomfortably close to our own. In order, therefore, to do effective work with couples, we need a setting in which we can be held not as clients, but as workers to our clients.

The psychodynamics of the interactive processes that we have discovered in working with couples in difficulties are to be found in all marriages and in all relationships. These processes are normal and healthy. They become pathological only in terms of the degree to which the patterns of interaction are adhered to by both partners, and the rigidity with which they do so, consciously and unconsciously.

We have come to see that the marriage relationship offers a unique opportunity for dealing with the unresolved conflicts of earlier relationships. The marital relationship offers scope for each partner to be parent and child to the other. With couples who can allow this to and fro between them without it threatening their adult and sexual selves, growth and development takes place without *too* much strain and stress. In such marriages each partner is certain enough of his own and the other's capacity for recovery—and each is certain enough of being held safe in the other's love.

Conflict is healthy, but its potential for growth is dependent upon the couple's capacity to regulate conflict in relation to their individual and shared internal worlds. This capacity to regulate conflict is itself possible only within a framework of a trustworthy defensive system. If a couple are going to risk discovering the real nature and quality of the conflicts within and between them, and if they risk getting painful feelings and anxieties located in the right places, then they will require a defensive system that is well tested and readily available, not demolished into fragments around their feet. Certain patterns of defensive interaction, agreed upon unconsciously by a couple, are established in the first place to defend against a shared fear (Bannister & Pincus, 1965).

In attempting to understand the rigidity of a defensive system operating between a couple, we start from the assumption that at some point in the *past* experience of each something has happened to make a defence necessary. The origin of that fear and anxiety—if it was ever consciously known—has long become hidden. In the marriage relationship, however, "it"—an often nameless dread—is related to as if it were always in the future: a catastrophe that has to be prevented at all costs, alongside a compulsive need to repeat it. The "catastrophe" is related to by the couple as if each is without adult resources to cope with it—giving a clue as to its origins. As one client put it: "I fear I will be like a small child falling with no one to catch me." The catastrophe that is so feared has already happened *and has been survived.* But perhaps it is not so much what happens to us as children that is so significant to future development, but how what happens is managed—whether there *is* someone there to catch you. Part of the purpose, perhaps, behind the compulsive need to repeat a past experience, to relive it, is to get in touch with the "original failure in the facilitating environment" (Winnicott, 1974), and from there to discover a better way of managing it in the present—a way that enhances growth and development, not stunts and cripples it.

Donald Winnicott, in his paper "Fear of Breakdown" (1974) written shortly before his death, gives birth to some of these ideas and takes them further by suggesting that "clinical fear of breakdown", or any other allied fear, is the "fear of a breakdown, *that has already been, but has not yet been experienced*". He considers that the "primary agony" has less to do with what happened and more to do with a sense of "nothing happening when something might profitably have happened". He suggests that the something that had already taken place could not be *experienced* because it happened at a time of "absolute dependency", before ego integration was mature enough to "encompass the experience", and that this experience is looked for compulsively in the future (Winnicott, 1974). I find this a very helpful and illuminating idea, and one that stimulates a further thought: that for some people the continuing attachment to and search for an unknown "something" might also have to do with the "something" ending before it had begun.

In therapy, two questions need eventually to be considered: (1) Is the rigidity of the defence, erected in the first place by a "small child with no one to catch him", still *so* necessary? (2) Can a couple risk finding out?

I find it helpful to think of a defensive system as a gate: if it is kept permanently closed, or always open, it fails in its purpose to facilitate growth and development. In therapy we do not seek to remove the gate, only to oil its hinges, allowing it both to open and shut, to help our clients towards a belief in themselves as their own gatekeepers.

The marriage relationship itself provides a kind of "container" in which the internal conflicts of each can be externalized and made accessible in the interactive processes the couple develop between them, keeping alive the hoped-for resolution of these conflicts, but within a defensive system that guards against the intolerable fears they are expected to arouse.

At the very core of every defensive system and of every emotional conflict lies the longing for a close intimate relationship with a significant other, and of being a self-sufficient "I"—independent, autonomous, certain of being able to survive alone. The longing, however, is associated with anxiety. For the longing for closeness arouses the fear of being "swallowed up", taken over, dominated by the other, leading to a loss of self. The longing for autonomy gives rise to fears of being abandoned, of being destructive, of survival threatened, and of the loss of the other. In the face of such conflict, ambivalence is born, and ways have to be found of managing loving and hating the same person.

* * *

A couple referred urgently by their general practitioner at a time of acute crisis were asked during the course of their initial consultation what had first attracted each to the other. I was struck by their replies and the language they used. She said it had been something to do with his "sense of freedom", and he that it was her "sense of security". I wondered about their history, and what it was that made the attractions for freedom for one and security for the other so compelling. The wife, Sally, had been brought up in a close-knit family unit in a small mining village in Northern England, "where everyone in the street was interrelated". The family had never been anywhere else. She told me that her upbringing had been very moral, and that her father had "strict views about things". The sense of being a family was valued more highly than was the

individual's growth and development within it. Nothing—
not her illegitimate pregnancy, nor her brother's
promiscuous homosexuality—was allowed to threaten the
family unit. Everything was drawn back into it and
encapsulated by what her husband Rodney described as
her parents' "bloody sensibleness".

Rodney's background was in sharp contrast to his wife's.
He was the younger of two sons, whose parents seemed
unable to risk their own tenuous relationship to include
the care and upbringing of their children. Rodney's older
brother was permanently cared for by foster parents with
whom he was evacuated during the war. Later, when
Rodney was born, his parents went to live next-door to the
foster parents, and a good deal of his caring was
undertaken by this couple. He described himself as a child
with two sets of parents, and that his childhood was a
constant struggle to keep in favour with both. When out of
favour with one set, he could always rely on being in
favour with the other.

So we have a couple attracted to each other but coming
from very contrasting backgrounds: his fragmented, with little
or no boundaries, hers close-knit, with boundaries rigidly maintained. In both, conflict is avoided, not regulated: in his, by running from one set of parents to the other, in hers, by everything
being "taken in". In terms of the "gate", his is kept permanently
open and hers permanently shut. No interchange, exchange, or
selection process was possible. Each thought they saw in the
other's experience that which they had so lacked in their own—
but the "security" that attracted him was experienced by her as
suffocation, and the "freedom" that she longed for was experienced by him as being abandoned and rootless. However, the
known, although unsatisfactory, is also familiar; anything outside experience, albeit attractive, is uncertain and fearful. Unconsciously, both the known and the not known are related to
ambivalently.

With such couples, each is trying to get from the other just
that very thing that the other is trying to get away from, therefore each confirming the other's worst fears that what they so
want and long for is also terrifying.

Like a great number of couples coming for help, Sally and Rodney experienced difficulties in finding a comfortable distance between each other. Closeness, although longed for, felt like a loss of self or being swallowed up by the other. But distancing, as when their baby arrived, felt like being lost to each other and abandoned. With this couple, the fear and the longing was too great to risk, regulating the conflict between their internal and external experience of "freedom" and "security". Instead, their marital interactions were a collusive defence against the extreme fears of both. I gained the impression of Sally sitting at home while Rodney was away working or in the pub, but being attached to her by a long umbilical cord. For a number of years, this was a reasonable compromise for them, although it did little towards promoting growth and development.

The crunch came, however, when his "freedom" and her "security" became too much for both. He had an affair and told Sally about it, promising to give the girlfriend up. She reacted by being "bloody sensible", and for the next two weeks they were very close, spending much of their time, day and night, in bed together. As a result Sally attempted to re-establish the "family unit" by becoming pregnant (with his help, of course). He then felt trapped into the marriage, but he thought that a baby would make them more separate and lost to each other. At the time of referral, he was threatening to leave Sally unless she had an abortion, and each described themselves as experiencing a "personality crisis".

Within this marriage relationship, each had discovered that behind their contrasting early experiences both shared a poor sense of personal identity, one of being insufficiently inside their own psychological skins to risk an intimate relationship.

Significantly, it is "not-good-enough" early relationships that are clung to by both parent and child, in spite of conscious wishes and actions to have it otherwise. People from such backgrounds often enter into marriage itself as a means of getting free of parents and leaving past experiences behind. They find, however, that unconsciously they have chosen a partner with whom they can repeat those earlier experiences, and the characteristic dynamics of the parent–child relationship become the dominating quality of their marital interaction. Failure to relinquish the parental relationship satisfactorily and its rediscovery in the marriage relationship is complex in its purpose. It attempts partially to deal with a shared guilt of each feeling "not good enough" for the other while keeping alive the hope that the "not good enough" will one day be transformed into that "ideal" relationship of their internal worlds—alongside which, of course, the reality will always feel to be "not good enough".

Idealization, and its opposite, denigration, is a defence against the consequences of ambivalence. The demand on the marriage relationship in such cases is to repeat the "not-good-enough" qualities of the primary relationship in order to transform it into the ideal. The more imperfect that early experience is felt to have been, the more the marriage relationship will be invested with idealized hopes and set up for the inevitable fall. Such couples often share a hatred for an "ordinary, good-enough relationship", and a pattern of "all or nothing" is a dominant feature of their interaction together.

I have spent some time in exploring the marriage relationship in its potential for defending against intolerable anxiety, guilt, and shame arising from conflict. If we turn the coin over, we see that the same marriage relationship is entered into with hope that the conflicts of the past and their expression in the present can be faced and dealt with; that commitment to an ordinary, good-enough relationship might be achieved and growth and development continued. For, far from being dull, flat, and lifeless, the "ordinary" is the middle ground between the "all and the nothing", where the creative tension between autonomy and intimacy, loving and hating, satisfactions and disappointment, having and not having can be regulated and creative potential can be realized.

With some couples, the *reality* of their past experiences is horrendous, and the marriage relationship is put under immense pressure to put the past right and/or to make it up to them by being something special. Most of us from time to time think life is unfair to us, and for some it *is* unfair. A woman who feels that life has treated her badly and owes her something may marry a man who has a compelling need to try to put things right. For other couples, however, it is less an acceptance of the *reality* of past experiences, and more a process of *restoring* that reality. For often the reality of the primary relationship has been seriously lost in the misperceptions and distortions brought about by one's own projections and the wish to see oneself and the other in a certain way.

A client of mine complained bitterly of his wife's rejection of him physically and sexually. He described his mother as having been totally rejecting of him in favour of his younger brother, but he could not recall any details of his childhood experiences. After leaving home, he developed physical symptoms whenever he visited her. In therapy, I experienced him as rejecting without thought everything I had to offer, often before I had completed a sentence. In accepting his view of things, we explored what was happening in the room with me in relation to how he experienced his wife and mother. This, however, did not bring any change, and he continued to reject everything I said, until I was having considerable difficulty in managing my exasperation. I wondered if rejecting me was related to his need to get in touch with the rejecting side of himself. This met with his usual response, but he went on to talk for the first time about a woman with whom he had lived for some time before meeting and marrying his wife. In describing this woman, he used exactly the same words he frequently used when telling me how he would like his wife to be towards him. When I asked what had happened to the relationship he replied, "I left her". He became distressed and said that when he got what he longed for, he could not stand it.

Over the next weeks I began to experience him differently; he no longer rejected everything I said, and he began to recall details of his childhood and adolescence. Together we began to question whether his long-held perception of how things were was entirely right. He sought out his mother, without suffering his usual physical symptoms, and checked things out with her. He learned that she had suffered considerable despair as to how to get through to this son who rejected every demonstration of her affection. In adulthood, he flew from a relationship that offered him warmth and closeness and married a woman who was *actually* totally rejected by her mother at birth.

In order to relinquish a relationship satisfactorily, it is necessary to know about one's attachment to it. Attachment to an important, but unsatisfactory and unreliable, person is often repressed and denied, or transformed into an idealized relationship, making it impossible for that relationship to be relinquished. The hope in its repeated experience in the marriage relationship is both to restore its reality and to discover the quality of one's attachment to it, in order for it then to be relinquished for growth and for maturation to continue.

With the couple just referred to, they shared an anxiety about being rejected and about managing their feelings in relation to this feared rejection. In her repeated rejection of her husband, the wife confirms his view of himself and of others, but at the same time carries and expresses for him the rejecting aspects of himself. The attachment to the relationship is carried firmly for both by him. Separation is constantly talked of and threatened, but never attempted. She has chosen a partner who, so long as she continues to reject him, will remain attached to her, reassuring her that she is, after all, loveable and wanted.

A further difficulty experienced in relinquishing an attachment to a perceived unsatisfactory parental relationship is the reluctance in "letting the parents off the hook". It involves unresolved anger with parents who are held responsible and blamed by their child for the dilemmas encountered in adult life. As a young woman put it, "if I get on with my life and make a go of it, my parents will feel they have done a good job—and they haven't. I want them to give me credit for having made a good job out of their bad one." Only slowly could she begin to recognize the enormous price she was paying for holding to this position and so begin to relinquish it. Paradoxically, as she did so, her relationship with her parents improved, and she also became more open to the possibilities and potential within her marriage.

This brings me to consider a further important aspect of the marriage relationship in its capacity to defend against anxiety and promote growth. People half-jokingly speak of their "better half" or "my other half". The marriage relationship provides a containment in which each feels the other to be a part of themselves—a kind of joint personality. What at first attracts and is later complained of in the other is often a projection of the disowned and frightening aspects of the self. It might be imagined that the best thing to do with unwanted aspects of the self is to project them onto someone or something and get as far removed as possible. That would, however, be placing a part of oneself in danger of being lost forever, and of losing one's potential for becoming a more complete person.

In unconsciously choosing a partner who for reasons of his own is willing to receive certain projections, it is possible to have unwanted aspects projected outside oneself and at the same time remain in vital contact with them in the other. What is projected into and rediscovered in the partner is then treated in the same way as it was treated in the self. What you cannot stand in yourself, you locate and attack (or nurture) in the other.

Because the one receiving the projection then carries a "double dose"—for example, his own angry feelings plus those of his partner—the feared aspect is in danger of becoming larger than life, confirming for both, albeit falsely, that it is really something to be terrified about. One partner might feel that certain feelings are frightening and totally unacceptable and be thankful that they do not belong to him and proceeds to attack them in the other. His partner, meanwhile, also receives confirmation that such feelings are terrifying but *is* thankful they are invested in her and thereby in her control. Frightening aspects of their "joint personality" are located in the partner who, both unconsciously agree, will best keep them safe and controlled.

A woman who severely controls in herself all expression of anger marries a man who can be easily provoked into violent outbursts in which he may break up furniture. There is evidence that although he appears to be out of control, he is never out of his own control and has never injured another person. We have in the therapy sessions reminded them both constantly of this fact. He has, however, married a woman he can rely upon to behave *as if* her own and especially their son's safety were threatened. Yet it is she, not he, who has in the past been violent to a child she was teaching. Just occasionally she confesses to murderous feelings and quickly disassociates herself from them, relying on her husband to express such feelings for both. He, on the other hand, can only feel safe if such feelings *are* in his control—his mother, father, and first wife met violent deaths.

Processes of projection and introjection go on in all marriages. Where the collusive system is reasonably flexible, and each partner feels safe enough inside his or her own skin and secure enough within the "containing skin" of their marriage relationship, both can feel free to explore in the other the projected aspects of themselves in order slowly to re-own them. Such a marriage is predominantly benevolent, each holding the other's interests at heart without outraging his own.

However, where this collusive system is rigidly maintained by both, as in the couple just mentioned, or where a move by one is countered by the other, the marriage relationship itself can at times of stress become severely threatened. Such couples may find their way into therapy seeking a safer container.

In therapy, the "inevitableness" of a couple's interaction is explored to discover its meaning—why it is as it is, and how it serves as both a constant preoccupation with a hidden dread and a defence against knowing about it. When gradually this hidden dread can be named and explored, it will often be discovered that the intense anxiety that lies behind it is shared by both, although the actual experience of each may be very different, sometimes seemingly the very opposite.

This intense and often crippling anxiety is always, I think, related to early loss and grief or shame and guilt, or a combination of each. Briefly, it involves anxiety in relation to what has happened or has been perceived to have happened to oneself, and secondly what the individual has done or perceived himself to have done to someone else.

The process of change itself involves the same loss and grief, shame, and guilt. However much change is wanted, it involves giving up the known for the unknown, the familiar for the unfamiliar, certainty for uncertainty. There are no guarantees, no assurances that there will be no further pain, or that others will not suffer in consequence. The alternative is to tiptoe through life, forever stepping back and turning aside from a living commitment to what *is*.

For some couples the hope for change is not possible and cannot be risked, because to do so feels, rightly or wrongly, to threaten life itself. Such couples agree unconsciously to live their lives together, relying on each other to maintain a defensive system that keeps hope alive, but forever around the next corner.

Some reach a point in their lives together when they can afford to lessen the defensive quality of their collusive interaction, only to find that change may be further resisted because of having to face the "wasted years". As one couple approaching their 60s remarked sadly, "if we could risk having things differently now, and we find it works for us, we have to face 30 wasted years".

Other couples are perhaps more courageous and can move towards facing the fact that for them no change is possible, and to experience grief, shame, and guilt in relation to the loss of hope itself. Paradoxically, at this very moment the process of change is begun. For growth starts from a recognition of where and what we are. Recognizing the past for what it is and accepting it as forever past releases one from the captivity of idealistic future hopes and enables one to begin to know where and what one is in the present. At this point we begin to discover what I like to name as the "great surprise of life". From the sad, angry, grief-stricken acceptance of where and what we are—involving acceptance of what cannot ever be and commitment to what is— we begin to experience a fulfilment and contentment that was previously thought possible only if the past could be made right and idealistic hopes obtained. Such is the process of transformation.

Perhaps, however, the most heroic and creative work of all lies in a willingness to question and explore the nature and quality of the interaction of the past with the present in order to transform both and leave the future free to create and become itself. Each time we enter a new experience with hope, we inevitably find someone or some circumstance in the immediacy of the new experience to provide a screen onto which we can project the terrors and hopes of our inner worlds. We find ourselves constantly on the alert for the flimsiest evidence on which to build and reconstruct our own old, old story.

It takes courage to face our terror of change and at the same time acknowledge our cherished attachment to our inner worlds and past experiences. However painful and distressful, however deep the depression that accompanies it, the repeated experience is welcomed with relief—for it is familiar, contains no surprises, is in our control—we know its lengths, depths, and breadths, and we have already survived it.

In the repeated experience, we allow the past to *take over* and consume the reality of the new experience in the present; it becomes *as if* the past were being relived. We see and relate to what is happening to us only in the light of the terrors and hopes of our inner worlds. It takes courage and energy to repeatedly ask oneself what the evidence is for such fears and hopes, and to acknowledge slowly that they are the makings of our own imaginings born of the dual need to keep things certain and in our control and to reach back to that which was "lost to begin with" and cannot now ever be.

When the past and the present are in relation to each other, each has the potential to act as a constraint—a brake on the other's strength, shaping and reshaping, influencing and being influenced, but without either's essential character and meaning being outraged. Like fire and water, each carries the potential to wipe the other out, but when in the right place and in relation to each other, their interaction produces steam, with all its potential for creativity and destruction. For there are no guarantees that the new experiences will be good or better than the old—only that they will be new and will take us forward.

Such are the processes that go on in a significant relationship between two people, such as in a marriage. Each partner brings to that relationship central aspects of their past experiences, established and nurtured within their inner worlds. In their interaction each has the potential to confirm the other's worst fears, and together they revisit the past experiences of each. But if these fears and perceptions can be challenged in the light of the evidence in their present external reality and be offered for exploration rather than for continued re-enactment, it becomes possible for the inner world of each and their shared outer world to be transformed.

A sculptor who holds within himself a certain image chooses a material that will best portray the essence of that image, and he allows this image to be influenced by the natural qualities of his chosen material. We are then invited to look upon, not the image or the material, but the magical potency of the interaction that took place between them and which transformed both, giving new meaning to each.

CHAPTER FIVE

Marriage
as a psychological container

Warren Colman

I have often wondered why it is that "long-term work" has a different meaning in marital psychotherapy from the one it has come to have in individual psychoanalytic psychotherapy. Nowadays it is not unusual for individual psychotherapy to extend over five years or more. Yet in my experience—and this applies to all the work done at the Tavistock Institute of Marital Studies—it is highly unusual for couples to continue in therapy beyond three years, and I know of only a handful of cases in the history of the unit that have gone on as long as five years. Yet our work is based on the same psychoanalytic principles and methods as those that inform individual therapy. Why should this difference exist, and what does it say about the differences between these two overlapping therapeutic approaches?

I would like to use this question of the differences between marital and individual therapy as an indication of what I take to be the defining feature of marital therapy—namely, that its aim is to promote the capacity of a marriage to function as a psychological container for the individuals within it. Sometimes, of course, it will become apparent in the course of therapy that this is not possible, and the work will then be about helping the

70

couple to separate. It does also happen that couples come for therapy having already decided to separate and wanting help to do so. Then it is a question of mourning the loss of the marital container or, at least, giving up the hope that it could be one. But in all cases I find it useful as a diagnostic aid to have in mind the question, is there a container, and if so, how is it functioning?

The fact that couples can—and do—separate points up an obvious difference between individual and marital therapy. For, although it could certainly be said that individual therapy also seeks to promote containment within the individual, there is no equivalent to the breakdown and separation of the container, which for the individual is tantamount to psychotic disintegration, whereas for the individuals in a couple it may be a healthy and fruitful outcome.

I take it as axiomatic that individuals require a sense of containment to be able to function creatively (and I shall be referring to what is meant by this later in the chapter). However, there are many arenas in which such containment may be found—work, religion, and artistic experience for example—and marriage is only one of these. Furthermore, the capacity to experience any of these as containing and, particularly, the quality of that containment—is it enabling or restrictive, for example—depends on the individual's own *internal* containment (integration). In that sense any external relationship such as marriage represents a symbolic realization of internal capacities, but, of course, this truth is reversible. External relationships *promote* internal capacities. This is the *raison d'être* of psychotherapy and, in its psychological function, of marriage too. Throughout this chapter I am concerned with the interaction of internal and external functioning, and therefore I draw on a comparison of marriage and psychotherapy as two kinds of "therapeutic institution", as well as looking at the difference between marital and individual therapy. Indeed, the fact that the therapy relationship between couple and therapist(s) is not the only potentially therapeutic relationship in the room during the course of marital psychotherapy is one of the major axes around which marital therapy revolves.

These considerations raise questions about treatment of choice. Given that the capacity to relate is an internal capacity and that for the marital therapist it is an external relationship that is the focus of treatment ("the patient is the marriage"), can marital therapy be done with couples who do not have in themselves a basic level of intra-personal integration and capacity for containment? If this capacity does not exist sufficiently, will the relationship the couple create between them be inadequate to provide material for the therapeutic endeavour? Some extremely disturbed individuals are capable of getting themselves married, but they may not have the basic capacity for relationship that the marital therapist normally takes for granted.

In practice, many such couples do get taken on for treatment. It is not so much a question of treatment of choice as a diagnostic issue. Such couples need a sort of "pre-therapy": a great deal of work must be done exploring the fundamental issues of what a relationship means. In my experience this requires far more attention to how the couple use the therapists than is necessary with most couples. By no means can it be taken for granted that these couples know what is meant by marital therapy, since they have precious little idea of what is meant by marriage. While I do believe that the couple focus does make it more difficult to get at the underlying disturbance, this may be precisely the reason why such people opt for marital therapy—individual therapy would be far too threatening. Similarly, many family therapists know that many problems that are presented through the children's difficulties are, fundamentally, marital problems, but to broach this too directly, too soon, would risk losing the family from treatment altogether. After nearly two years of marital therapy, one husband said to me, "I have *no* problems, no problems whatever—my only problem is *her*". This is not always his attitude, but it clearly demonstrates that there are occasions when therapy is threatening enough for this man to require the presence of his wife as a receptacle for his evacuated "problems".

I have already referred to the maxim, "the patient is the marriage". This implies that the focus of marital therapy is on what the couple create between them, the relationship itself, rather than the internal world of the individuals. This does not mean that the internal world is not considered—far from it—but it does mean that the arena in which it is revealed and explored is the marital relationship, and that those aspects of the internal world that appear in the transference between couple and therapist also, by definition, refer to the marriage. For whereas the individual therapist deliberately conducts himself in such a way as to reduce to a minimum the limitations of what can be brought into the transference, the partners in a marriage are continually defining between them the limits of what can be expressed within the relationship, such that the "material" that is brought to the therapy is, in a sense, pre-defined. It bears the shape of, indeed is the psychic expression of, the couple's interaction. In other words, whereas the individual therapist's focus is on the internal world *per se* and he addresses himself to the interaction between himself and the patient in order to reveal this, the marital therapist's focus is on the interaction between the couple *as an end in itself*. Where he addresses himself to the transference, his interventions are geared to revealing aspects of the marital interaction rather than the separate individual internal worlds that comprise it. He is, indeed, concerned with the couple's *shared* internal world, but I think it is important to recognize that individuals are too complex and multi-faceted for the whole of their psychic life to find expression within a marital relationship—however central in their lives that relationship may be.

This is, in fact one of the most fundamental tensions in marriage—between the autonomous development of the individuals and their allegiance to the shared world of the partnership. Acceptance of the fact that this tension can never be dissolved is, therefore, one of the major disillusionments that each couple has to negotiate on the way to establishing a satisfactory relationship, which provides "good-enough" containment. Here again there is a difference between the individual and the marital focus. For, whereas the individual's drive to wholeness, or individuation, aims (ideally) at an ever more encompassing containment of psychic contents within an integrated self, this would not be a desirable aim for a marital container even if it were possible. Rather, the marital container must, paradoxically, be able to contain the tension that arises from the need of the individuals to develop outside the relationship as well as within it. For to be totally contained within a relationship would require the abolition of separateness and individual autonomy—the very opposite of individuation.

Returning to the question with which I began: it used to be believed that the relative brevity of marital therapy suggested that it might be a more effective form of treatment than individual therapy. Like so much of the therapeutic optimism that flourishes in the initial enthusiasm of new developments, this view does, I think, need to be revised in the light of the foregoing considerations. It is not that it is more effective in general, but that it is effective in a specific, more limited, and less thoroughgoing area. It is certainly true that the mutually reinforcing nature of marital projections can preserve the status quo against the most zealous efforts of an individual therapist, but this is only to make the diagnostic point that in such cases marital therapy should perhaps be the treatment of choice. For it is also true that a good outcome of marital therapy may be that one partner seeks individual therapy.

Clinical illustration:
Mr and Mrs Blake

Mr and Mrs Blake sought treatment for an infertility problem that had been diagnosed as psychological. Mrs Blake duly conceived after the initial consultation, and we continued to work with them throughout the pregnancy. The area of difficulty proved to be a number of miscarriages several years earlier, culminating in the premature birth of a child who died while still in intensive care. These losses rebounded for Mrs Blake on a difficult relationship with her mother, in which she felt repeatedly abandoned, and, for Mr Blake, on the actual abandonment by his mother, who had died in his early childhood. Neither of them had been able to grieve, both were wracked by guilt, and each was terrified of the reflection in the other of the enormity of their own unmet needs for mothering. These anxieties, their shared phantasy, issued in an interaction in which Mrs Blake became the damaged baby/mother whom Mr Blake endlessly but resentfully attempted to repair—their shared defence (Clulow, Dearnley, & Balfour, 1986). We were able to help them considerably over the period of the pregnancy, and once the new baby had safely weathered the early weeks and remained healthy, they decided to end their therapy. They returned, however, some months later, with Mrs Blake in the grip of a near-psychotic depression.

Although this did recede and the couple's relationship stabilized, both as partners and as parents, it had now become apparent that Mrs Blake's anxieties about rejection and abandonment were more deep-rooted than her husband's. They were embedded in the overall quality of the mothering she received in infancy and in her internal phantasy life, whereas her husband had been faced by a more concrete event in childhood, which he was now able to "place" and mourn. He was relieved of the need to care for his wife compulsively, and she was thereby freed to seek individual therapy for herself. Although Mrs Blake clearly needed further help, we felt it was important to work towards a final ending of the marital therapy, since to have continued would have been to collude with their fears that separations were inevitably disastrous and therefore could not be tolerated. At the last session Mr Blake said, "we still have the same problems, only now we are able to talk about them". Perhaps this was because they had also been helped to recognize that within their own relationship they were separate people, with separate difficulties, as well as those they shared. Now that this recognition did not need to be so rigidly defended against, both partners felt safe enough to allow each to follow their own path. They did not *both* (or neither) have to have therapy.

Comment:
positive and negative therapeutic containment

Mr Blake's summing-up serves as a good description of the achievement of a satisfactory marital container. When they left us, Mr and Mrs Blake were not a very happy couple, and they still had a great many difficulties, but we nevertheless felt that as *marital* therapists we had taken them as far as it was possible for them to go at that time. We had been able to provide a temporary container, which the couple had used to rely on while a necessary re-orientation took place in the marriage. The transition from the couple twosome to becoming a threesome was fraught with danger for this couple, as for many others, and either in prospect or retrospect is one of the major crises impelling couples to seek help (Clulow, 1982).

Although the not-often-exceeded two to three years of marital psychotherapy, as mentioned earlier, is somewhat arbitrary, and is certainly no more than a rule of thumb, it is, I think, to do with the temporary nature of the marital therapy container. It is as though the therapeutic container is "borrowed" over a transitional period and needs to be discarded relatively quickly, before the couple's capacity to use their own relationship in a therapeutic way becomes atrophied or, as sometimes happens, the therapy sessions become the *only* place where that capacity can be exercised. Looked at the other way round, couples usually want therapy to end around this time, perhaps because the containment is more easily integrated into an existing relationship, as opposed to the individual patient's need either to adapt his existing relationships or to create new ones. The individual's achievement is, however, perhaps more flexible and adaptable: he or she is like the artisan who owns his own tools, whereas the recipients of marital therapy are more like the industrial worker who uses the tools provided by the factory (i.e. the marriage).

There are various alternative scenarios to the positive use of the therapy as a temporary container that can result in therapy going on endlessly, although they are not primarily to do with the length of therapy, but with the way it is used. The subject requires a separate chapter but I will mention here two situations in which the therapist(s) may become embroiled in a unconscious collusive impasse. Often the process is a subtle one and requires particularly close scrutiny of the countertransference. Resentment, boredom, and frustration in the therapist are often indications that something is amiss in the way therapy is being used, although these affects may, of course, have other sources.

It may be, for example, that there is an underlying hatred of relationship in the couple, associated especially with envy and the intolerance of need to which it gives rise. This can be subtly re-enacted in the transference to the therapist(s) who can soldier on for years, like Penelope's suitors, unaware that all the gains of the day are unpicked again by night.

An alternative scenario, and one that I have encountered more often, is that there is really no longer a marriage to "save" (if there ever was), and the couple are using the therapy to prevent their having to face up to this. The containment provided by the therapeutic relationship may then be used as a *substitute* for the containment that was sought, and not found, in the marriage. This is a very different matter from using the therapy as a "temporary container" to rely on while a necessary re-orientation takes place in the marriage.

This last point brings me to an important complication in my argument. Therapy, whether individual or marital, not only seeks to *promote* containment, but it also *provides* it as one of its main functions. Before going on to give a clinical example of containment in marital therapy, I need to state more clearly what is meant by this idea, since, like many semi-technical terms in psychoanalytic usage, containment is used in a number of overlapping but distinguishable ways. It is, in fact, more often used in this second sense of being part of what the therapist offers—or should offer—to his patients. Containment is part of a model that is both drawn from and read back into the mother–infant relationship. Bion, with whom I shall begin, uses the concept explicitly, but I shall also refer to other closely related concepts, such as Winnicott's ideas on "holding", because these ideas are also closely related to the sense in which marriage can be said to function as a container.

Bion:
container/contained

Bion's model of the container/contained derives from his enquiry into the origins of thinking. He sought to explain deficiencies in the capacity for learning from experience in terms of a mental function he named "alpha function" and which he purposely left undefined (Bion, 1962a). He believed that this capacity needed to be developed in the infant through the initial relationship with the mother, who plays, as Donald Meltzer has described it, a pedagogical role (Meltzer, 1988).

The mother's function is to contain those aspects of her infant's experiences—particularly bad experiences—that the infant elicits in her via his projective identification. In due course, if she is emotionally available to her infant, she is able to process these projections and to make sense of them by means of her "reverie". They then become available for re-introjection by the infant in a modified, more tolerable form (Bion, 1962b). Eventually, Bion suggests, the function of containment becomes installed in the infant and forms the basis for the development of alpha function. Thus, to begin with, the mother is the container and the infant the contained; later, the container/contained forms an internal apparatus within the child's own psyche.

Bion's model provides a clear account of how, in psychotherapy, the provision of containment by the therapist promotes containment in the patient. The therapist's "evenly suspended attention" is the equivalent of the mother's "reverie". He gives back to the patient, via his interpretations, those psychic elements he has been able to process, thus promoting the patient's capacity to think about and to reflect upon his own experience. The end of analysis is when the patient has developed the capacity for self-analysis—when, ideally, he has internalized the analytic function and the external analyst can be discarded. The institution of psychotherapy, unlike the institution of marriage, is intended as a temporary one, and its success is demonstrated (at least, in part) by its dissolution.

The analytic container

Bion's model of the container/contained is often equated with the idea of analysis or therapy being itself a containing environment, although Bion's usage is really more specific, referring to a particular function that the analyst may fulfil for the patient. The idea of analysis offering a container *per se* is more to do with the structure of the analytic setting, the analyst's commitment to maintaining a consistent *frame*. The features that make up the frame are such things as regularity of sessions,

protection from interruptions and intrusions, and the consistency of the analytic attitude. The issue here is essentially one of
boundaries: the analyst takes responsibility for maintaining
boundaries both around and within the relationship with the
patient, and these boundaries make up the container. They
create a space within which analytic work is possible. If the
space is disturbed, then so are the delicate processes at work
within it.

Marion Milner has described the frame as marking off a
different kind of reality. As she says, "it is the existence of this
frame that makes possible the full development of that creative
illusion we call transference" (Milner, 1955). Jung, drawing on
the symbolism of alchemy, compared analysis to the alchemist's *vas hermeticum*, the sealed vessel. Furthermore, he compared the development of the transference to the alchemist's
symbolic representations of the processes taking place within
the *vas* in terms of the *marriage* of the King and Queen (Jung,
1946). This is reminiscent of Bion's algebraic notation of the
container/contained, for which he used the signs for male and
female, ♂♀, the female containing the male (Bion, 1962a). In
Donald Meltzer's work on beauty and creativity, the source
of inspiration is described as the "nuptial chamber" (Meltzer,
1988).

These symbolic images should not be confused with the
reality of marriage in the external world, but they do demonstrate that the idea of containment forms part of the archetypal
base, the psychic pre-conception of the marriage relationship
and, vice versa, that marriage is a highly appropriate representation for symbolizing processes of containment.

Winnicott:
holding

A number of attempts have been made to compare Bion's concept of containment with Winnicott's ideas about "holding".
Some authors (for example, Shuttleworth, 1989) hardly distinguish between the two; others (for example, James, 1984) insist
that they are quite different, while having close links.

Both theories refer to aspects of the mother–infant relationship on the one hand and the psychoanalytic situation on the
other. However, Winnicott and Bion arrived at their theories
from quite different perspectives, or "vertices", to use Bion's
word. This does, I think, go some way to explaining the different
emphases, although in practice it is often very difficult to distinguish whether any particular event would be best described
as holding or containment. After all in the original mother–
infant situation it is ultimately the same range of phenomena
being described.

While Bion's ideas about mothering were drawn from the
psychoanalysis of adults, Winnicott drew heavily on his life-
long experiences as a paediatrician, observing real mothers
with real infants. He applied these observations to his work as
a psychoanalyst—the exact reverse of Bion's approach. It is
therefore not surprising that Bion tends to see mothers as be-
having rather like a kind of analyst, whereas Winnicott tends to
see analysts as needing to behave, at least in part, rather like a
kind of mother. Bion's notion is of a much more explicitly active
process—the mother who receives, processes, and returns the
infant's projections. Winnicott's emphasis is, rather, on the
mother who *allows* her infant to discover his own inner being in
his own way and in his own time. Her role is a protective one,
managing the situation by means of her emotionally reliable
presence, so that the infant can safely experience total dependence, sufficiently free of impingements that he does not need to
develop premature ego functions (Winnicott, 1960a).

It is important to recognize that Winnicott's main interest
was in *normal* developmental processes, while Bion's theories
were an attempt to understand disturbances of psychotic pro-
portions. However, it should not be thought that Winnicott's
suggestion is of a passive process, with the infant doing all
the work. Clearly, the mother needs to be extremely actively
involved in providing just the right kind of adaptation for the
infant. In its application to the analytic situation holding may
include the interpretation of the patient's deepest anxieties
(Winnicott, 1963b). What Winnicott does not do, however, is to
describe the processes going on within the mother, or the analyst's mind: the working of projective identification. Furthermore, where the original maternal process has failed, the need

for holding and containment—the provision of a secure environment and the processing of projections—is dramatically increased and it is these situations of failure that crop up in the consulting room and in disturbed marriages.

Having described the main references to containment in the analytic relationship and the way this interacts with images of the mother-infant relationship, I now want to introduce some more detailed clinical material. The example I shall give illustrates the way the provision of containment in the therapy relationship can ultimately promote containment of the kind that is appropriate to marriage. I leave aside until later the discussion of the nature of the marital container.

Mr and Mrs Hall

Mr and Mrs Hall sought marital therapy due to a crisis that had been precipitated in the marriage by Mr Hall having an affair. They had each briefly sought individual therapy but had not found this helpful, and they felt that it was the marriage that needed attention, although Mr Hall was still deeply uncertain whether he wished to remain in it. The affair, however, had apparently now come to an end.

Mr Hall's complaint was that his wife was distant, unaffectionate, and sexually disinterested. He was also critical of her mothering of their 3-year-old son, whom Mrs Hall had virtually abandoned to the care of nannies and other helpers. Mrs Hall showed little direct feeling but described being bewildered by the sudden disruption to what she had taken to be a happy, untroubled marriage. Mr Hall had always been frequently away from home on business, but this had brought them a luxurious and exciting lifestyle that Mrs Hall very much enjoyed. She did not miss him when he was away. In the sessions her demeanour was detached and unemotional, and both therapists experienced her as remote.

When marital therapy began, Mrs Hall was 6 months pregnant—she had conceived at the time they had first decided to seek therapy. Mr Hall was extremely

preoccupied throughout the first few sessions about
whether, in view of the pregnancy, this was the right time
to engage in therapy. He was clearly worried about
damaging either his wife, the unborn child, or both, if he
exposed all his doubts about the marriage. Mrs Hall,
however, sought to persuade him of her robustness.

We knew from the assessment (which had been made by a
colleague) that Mrs Hall was an only child whose mother
had lost two babies subsequent to her—one at eight
months pregnant, the other at a few months old—but we
found ourselves unable to comment on this. Our response
to Mr Hall's uncertainty was to suggest that, instead of
worrying about whether they should "go into all this", as
Mr Hall put it, they should "just come". This suggestion
was greeted with relief, and the sessions became markedly
less tense. In effect, we were offering to provide a
temporary containment at a period when they were unable
to contain the unconscious anxieties about whether they
might destroy the unborn child. At this point, however, we
were only aware of these issues theoretically, as it were.
We were offering an environment that *could* contain, akin
therefore to holding, and inviting projections that we would
have to contain, in Bion's sense.

In retrospect it is possible to see that Mrs Hall had
projected the anxieties she could not contain into her
husband, but he was unable to contain them either. Even
his affair may have been a response to this unconscious
pressure, a desperate attempt to seek containment outside
the marriage. If Mrs Hall unconsciously believed that she
was responsible for the death of her mother's subsequent
babies, this might well account for her fear of getting close
to anyone she loved, especially her husband and child.
The imminent arrival of a second child—the event that had
never successfully been negotiated by her own mother—
had brought that anxiety to a head.

These anxieties were never taken up directly in the
therapy, but, to our surprise, this did not seem necessary
to the couple's considerable improvement. The baby was

due over the Christmas holiday—the first break in the therapy. At the last session before Christmas Mr Hall told us he had suffered a near-fatal blood clot to his heart two days previously, but it had dispersed just in time! Mrs Hall laughed hysterically as her husband drolly recounted his colleagues' dumbfoundedness when he had abruptly abandoned an important business meeting to go to the hospital. I commented that he was telling us that he was afraid that the situation he was in was killing him. We were also sufficiently concerned to arrange for a colleague to be available if the couple needed to be seen over the break. We were now "in business" as a holding environment, our response arising out of a countertransference of concern that we hardly questioned, so syntonic was it to their needs.

As we had heard nothing from them, we assumed that the baby had not yet arrived by the time we resumed in the New Year. In fact, the baby had been born six days previously, but an extremely well-looking Mrs Hall arrived in high spirits for the first session—without the baby. When I saw her, I was overwhelmed by the fantasy that she had got rid of it—it was not in her tummy, and it was not in her arms, so where was it? While my co-therapist engaged with the couple's delight, I sat shocked and silent for almost the whole session. Eventually I was able to link what I was feeling to Mrs Hall's childhood experience of her mother's baby, which must have disappeared in exactly this way in the eighth month of pregnancy. I did not feel able to speak to this link directly but was able to enquire about the baby's absence.

In subsequent sessions Mrs Hall was able to get in touch with feelings of remorse and regret for the way she had virtually abandoned her first child, stimulated by the experience of having made a more successful bonding with the new baby. The change in her style of mothering was minimal, however, as she still preferred to leave most of the baby's care to others and was noticeably "unmaternal". It was difficult to imagine her as capable of "reverie", and it is intriguing that in the therapy it was I who had the reverie about the missing baby, not my female co-therapist. This reflected the dynamics of the marriage, where Mr Hall was the more emotional, reflective, and introspective of the two. My experience was a registration in the countertransference of the force with which Mrs Hall had unconsciously projected her anxieties into her husband.

The couple continued in therapy only a further six months after the birth of the baby. They reported considerable improvement in their relationship, finding themselves able to communicate more openly and share more enjoyment than they had done for years. Significantly, we were not told, and did not enquire, about their sexual relationship. Mr Hall made important changes in his attitude to his career, feeling less driven and perfectionistic. Towards the end, Mrs Hall, having been the more reluctant partner, became openly valuing of the therapy and said that when they first came, nothing was certain in their lives except the regularity of the sessions—an explicit valuing of the structural aspect of containment. Mr Hall had described his affair as being like the violent springing-out of a "Jack-in-the-box". It seemed that the "Jack" was now more securely contained and, while they may have still needed to keep the lid on it, a crucial advance had been made in that their anxieties about death and annihilation had been contained.

The success of the therapeutic work was due to the focus we took—not the one that was initially presented, Mr Hall's affair, but the anxiety over producing a second child. Thus my dramatic countertransference experience when I felt that Mrs Hall had got rid of the baby was the crucial turning point. This was the unconscious shared fantasy that was too explosive for the couple to contain (Meltzer, 1982) and required an outside agency to prevent the disintegration, not so much of the individuals, as of the couple itself. The "Jack-in-the-box" symbolized this beautifully: whether it represents the destructive baby in the womb or the destructive ejaculating penis, it is an image of dangerous and aggressive sexuality.

For Mrs Hall this would be the destructive parental inter-course, which produced dead or damaged babies. For Mr Hall there was a corollary to this: at the age of 15 he had felt suicidal after discovering that his girlfriend was pregnant. The child was born, but Mr Hall has never had any contact with either the child or the mother.

In describing our work with Mr and Mrs Hall, I have referred to the key moments in which holding and containment were provided by the therapists. It is apparent that one cannot really operate without the other, since it was by virtue of our struc-ture and our reliable presence that we were able to contain the forceful projection of their "destroyed baby" fantasy. By our understanding and tolerance of it, the couple were able to re-ceive it back detoxified, even though it was still, for them, largely unconscious. I believe this is what Winnicott means by the analyst's survival. It is not enough simply to carry on being there—what is at issue is the therapists' living presence, their survival as a "thinking object".

I would now like to move on to a discussion of the kind of containment we promoted in their marriage. I shall continue to use material from Mr and Mrs Hall's therapy to illustrate the ways in which the containing function of marriage has been described by other writers, especially Janet Mattinson (Mattin-son & Sinclair, 1979; see also Lyons & Mattinson, chapter six, this volume).

Defensive containment
and Jung's container/contained

Prior to Mr Hall's affair, the Halls' marriage exemplified a *de-fensive* form of containment. Outside the analytic world, con-tainment is frequently referred to in this way—for example, the police "containing" a riot. In this defensive sense containment is a way of keeping those outside the container safe from what is within it, sealing off a problem, rather than creating a space within which to work at it.

Mattinson and Sinclair have described the purpose of de-fensive containment in marriage as being,

to ward off conscious and unconscious anxieties of both
partners and to prohibit development. We have found that
often these anxieties are shared, so that both partners have
the same vested interest in trying to avoid particular situations that they feel might be disastrous. [Mattinson &
Sinclair, 1979]

For Mr and Mrs Hall it was necessary to maintain considerable emotional distance to prevent anxieties about guilt, loss,
and destructiveness from emerging. Mr Hall had almost consciously chosen the unemotional Mrs Hall as being very different from his own emotionally overwhelming mother, who
seemed to have used him as her narcissistic object (Miller,
1983) and whose demands for high achievement he had felt it
incumbent on him to meet. Both, therefore, had a vested interest in not becoming too entangled with the other, albeit for
somewhat different reasons.

More subtly, however, Mr Hall found himself back in the
same old role. He resented the demands of his high-flying career and felt that it was more for Mrs Hall's benefit than his
own, since she was the one who expected the luxurious lifestyle
it provided. Similarly, behind the cool independence of the Mrs
Hall who did not miss her husband when he was away, there
was a more childlike woman, who was completely dependent on
her husband, with little sense of her own separateness. This
was shown up by the depth of her shock when Mr Hall's affair
was revealed.

Jung, as long ago as 1925, described this sort of marriage
as the problem of the container and the contained (Jung,
1925). Mrs Hall was wholly contained by her husband, but Mr
Hall found that the marriage worked on him, as Jung puts it,
"like a room that was too small", and he found himself "spying
out of the window". As I have suggested, the increased unconscious demands from Mrs Hall for her husband to contain her
anxieties about her capacity to mother brought matters to a
head by overloading the defensive arrangement. Mr Hall became acutely aware that he was not being emotionally (or sexually) contained, and he turned to another woman.

Jung's model of the container/contained should not be
confused with the idea of marriage as a container (let alone

Bion's container/contained). On the contrary, it is more like that which the Halls demonstrate: a defensive arrangement, and ultimately an unstable one. Rather than the *relationship* acting as a container, there is an attempt to make one *partner* the container for the other, and this almost inevitably results in "spying out of the window", with the containing partner desperately seeking his/her own containment outside the marriage. Of course, this does not always take the form of an extra-marital affair—it may equally lead one partner into individual therapy.

The container/contained marriage is rooted in an anti-developmental collusion, whereby one partner is able to remain a child and is spared the need to internalize the container/contained apparatus, while the other partner participates vicariously in this. [Lyons and Mattinson (chapter six, this volume) have pointed out that the conscious container is often the unconscious contained.] Mrs Hall's lack of emotional involvement was shared by her parents. She had no memories of her mother having grieved or been depressed by her losses, and the likelihood is that Mrs Hall had received the same sort of mothering that she provided for her first child. In other words, she had not been contained herself and sought this in a defensive way through her own marriage. She continued to use splitting, denial, and projection as her means of defence, and her husband found himself on the receiving end of her unmanageable projections.

Marriage as a therapeutic institution

In much of the literature on marriage its potentiality as a therapeutic institution is stressed. Defensive marriages are contrasted with developmental ones, where, to quote Lyons and Mattinson, the marriage provides "a container which will give (the partners) room in which to be, and (provides) for the expression of instinctual drive and feeling so that they may further their development and come to know more fully the different parts of themselves, eventually getting these parts into a more satisfying conjunction" (chapter six, this volume).

I would like to explore this statement by returning to the comparison between marriage as a therapeutic institution and the institution of therapy. To my mind this points up the boundaries of the marital container by showing what it is not. I believe that many couples who come for therapy have been unconsciously attempting to use their partners as though they were therapists and have inevitably got into difficulties when it turned out they were not. This is especially the case in the container/contained type of marriage.

It should be readily apparent that marriage cannot provide the same conditions for development—or, more precisely, re-development—as are available via psychotherapy. The therapist–patient relationship is, like the mother–infant relationship, an asymmetrical one, in which one partner takes responsibility for providing containment for the other. This allows for possibilities of regression that no other relationship, however intimate, can safely offer. In a marriage each partner needs to retain some awareness of his or her responsibility to the other, at the same time as enjoying the opportunities for regression that the relationship provides (Lyons, chapter ten, this volume). No marriage can withstand the sort of demands that even an averagely neurotic analytic patient may need to make on an analyst. In fact, by the use of the couch and the contained freedom of the analytic situation, patients are encouraged to regress in order that, in Michael Fordham's phrase, "the primary entities may be reached" (Fordham, 1978). By virtue of his own training and analysis, the analyst is "experienced" in Bion's rather specialized use of the word and able to contain those elements of the patient's experience that have previously been uncontained (Bion's beta elements), so that they become available for processing into the raw material of thought (Bion, 1962a).

Apart from the excessive demands that are required for one marital partner to contain another in this way—one thinks of the complaint that many wives make about their husbands, once they become mothers, of having two babies to look after—the very fact that couples choose each other on the basis of shared unconscious anxieties indicates that each will have the greatest difficulty containing the other precisely in those areas where they need containment most. Residual beta elements can only be dealt with defensively or by seeking a container outside the marriage. The mindless repetition of many marital rows suggests that they, and other similar difficulties, are the outcome of undigested beta elements ricocheting between the partners as each tries more and more urgently to lodge the projection into the other. In fact, when one partner does succeed in containing the other in an asymmetrical way, so that the contained partner grows and develops through the relationship, the marriage frequently turns out to be the casualty, since the erstwhile contained finds that he or she has outgrown the relationship. In short, marriage may be therapeutic, but it is not therapy. This is another and perhaps the most crucial aspect of the disillusion that each couple has to negotiate as they come to realize that some of the developmental hopes on which they may have based their marriage are bound to be disappointed. However, in couples who have past experience of being able to manage loss and disappointment, this realization will itself prove capable of containment.

Jung was intuitively well aware of this. He described how the breakdown of the container/contained arrangement initiates the demand for individuation in each of the partners and how each needs to find an inner integration before a truly psychological relationship becomes possible (Jung, 1925).

The marital container

The primary limitation of the defensive container/contained marriage is that, at best, only one partner is contained by the relationship, with the other functioning as a pseudo-therapist, while, at worst, the containment functions to deposit projections in a way that, it is hoped, will control them but does not modify them. Certainly a more flexible arrangement is when each partner can at times contain the other on a sort of "taking turns" basis, but this requires something more than a simple reversal. It demands a shift in the image each partner has of the relationship. The *relationship itself* becomes the container, the creative outcome of the couple's union, to which both partners can relate. It is an image of something the couple are

continually in the process of creating, sustaining, and maintaining, while at the same time feeling that they exist within it—
are contained by it. When couples talk of "our relationship", it
is this image they refer to—something that is felt to exist inde-
pendently of them and yet to which both are required to contribute. "The relationship" is like a third party—the symbolic
child—albeit the child may be conceived as a blessing or a
curse, the fruit of creative or of destructive intercourse.

I expect the reader will have noticed that both the couples I
have used to provide clinical illustrations of containment in
marital therapy produced a baby during the course of therapy
and that in both cases anxieties over the meaning of that baby
were central to their difficulties. If so, the reader is more aware
than I was when I first chose these examples. Although this is
indeed a fairly frequent occurrence in the course of marital
therapy, I suspect the unconscious significance of my choice
has more to do with the child as the symbolic representation of
any creative intercourse—that is, the outcome of the union of
container and contained, the meeting of King and Queen in the
alchemical *vas hermeticum* referred to earlier.

Marital therapy is primarily directed towards this shared
internal image of the relationship, which is essentially an image
of the couple in intercourse: the container is actually the total
"container/contained apparatus" (Bion, 1962a). The changes
that occur in the couple refer not so much to changes in the
individuals, but to a change in the quality of their relationship.
Through allowing the therapist(s) to participate in their interaction, its nature is altered, and a different image of relationship
becomes available for introjection. The work that the therapists
do in containing the relationship—thinking about it and sharing that thinking—is equivalent to a process of projection and
re-introjection in modified form. But the point I want to stress
is that the modified projections are re-introjected directly into
the couple's experience of the relationship. It is academic
whether the external interaction changes before the internal
images or vice versa, since internal and external are in continual interaction anyway; probably sometimes one, sometimes
the other predominates. But the marital therapist does have at
his or her disposal an important resource that the individual

therapist does not—a real external relationship other than the patient-therapist transference relationship.

The suggestion here is that the container/contained apparatus referred to by Bion somehow exists *between* the couple as well as being internal to each. At first I had difficulty in believing that there could be an equivalent for Bion's conception of the container within a two-person system. As I saw it, alpha function referred to an intra-psychic process and was intimately linked with an experiencing consciousness. Since marriage in itself does not possess either of these qualities, I could not see how it could itself be a container, in the sense of processing phenomena. However, the same conceptual difficulty would apply to the idea of an "introjection into the relationship". It then occurred to me that alpha function is an unconscious process, and if it makes sense to speak of shared unconscious fantasies, why shouldn't some kind of experience-processing function also form part of a couple's shared unconscious? What the couple in fact share is an unconscious image of a relationship in which male and female mate. If this is conceived of as a fruitful intercourse, then some creative outcome must result. Marital therapy, especially in a foursome, has its impact on this shared image, but this shared image must in turn affect the individual's own internal marriage—their nuptial chamber, as Meltzer describes it (Meltzer, 1988).

This, I believe, is the source of the enhanced integration that marriage can produce and that is referred to in the notion of the developmental marriage. Although, as I said earlier, the level of the individuals' integration will set limits to what the marriage can contain, the experience of actual intercourse can stimulate some development of an internal intercourse, provided the shared image of a parental couple is not too frightening and does not have to be too rigidly defended against. This is why, as Mattinson discovered in her work with mentally handicapped couples, some very limited individuals function better together than they do apart (Mattinson, 1970). Thus the development in Mr and Mrs Hall was from an image of destructive intercourse, symbolized by dead and aborted babies, to a more creative one, symbolized by the healthy second child and enacted in the therapy. The destructive "Jack" was still contained in the box, but by a more flexible repression, rather than by splitting and denial. This formulation correlates with Bion's elaboration of alpha function as providing the condition for a division in the mind between conscious and unconscious (Bion, 1962a).

The point here is that what in individual therapy must be internalized as a symbolic union of male and female can, in marital therapy, be left partially externalized. The couple rely on each other to provide a shared image of mating on which each of them can then draw. But what is required for this to be effective is some capacity to tolerate separateness and difference. For only two individuals who are separate and different can come together to create a fruitful intercourse. Naturally this is symbolized by and usually enacted through the sexual difference of male and female. It is not my intention, however, to exclude from homosexual relationships, of which I have very little knowledge, the possibility of fruitful and creative intercourse.

There are, of course, further conditions for the creation of an effective marital container, and these relate to the other senses of containment referred to earlier in the chapter. Intercourse alone, whether purely sexual or in its original, more generalized sense, is clearly not enough to make a marriage. There also needs to be a commitment to the relationship, providing for each of the partners a sense of trust, security, and reliability. Marriage then can become, in Winnicott's phrase, a holding environment. Similarly, it represents for most people the adult form of attachment.

In *Mate and Stalemate*, a study of work undertaken in a Social Services Department with couples who presented intractable marital difficulties, Mattinson and Sinclair (1979) drew heavily on attachment theory to explain the apparently self-defeating, often paradoxical behaviour of the couples they saw. They clarify the link between containment and attachment when they say, "Just as a young child needs to be contained and given a base from which to explore and to which to retreat, so too may an adult develop more of his fullness of nature if provided with an emotional container".

In our work with couples experiencing some disturbance in their relationship, it is often necessary to trace the point at which development has become blocked by the couple's shared defences in order that the couple may experience, in Lyons and Mattinson's phrase, "a more satisfying conjunction between the parts of themselves" (chapter six, this volume). However, this active developmental process in which marriage enables "the putting right of what was felt to be wrong" (Balint, chapter two, this volume) is only one side of the coin and the view from marital therapy is therefore skewed in certain respects. For, as well as promoting growth, marriage also needs to promote stability, and this creates a further tension within the relationship. Some couples may complain of stagnation, but for others the complaint may be of living in a state of permanent crisis. In the case of Mr and Mrs Hall, there had been a violent swing, precipitated by Mr Hall's affair, from the one to the other.

A more healthy state—if it is permissible to make such a recommendation for the infinite variety of workable arrangements that couples make—is a container that is flexible enough to allow for the inevitable transitions that every couple must experience, but also stable enough to *protect* them from too much of the anxiety that continual change creates. Development needs to be understood as a natural process of unfolding and adaptation to the changes inherent in the life-cycle. This should be distinguished from re-development in the sense of the re-working of infantile conflicts. Like all major life transitions, the formation of a committed partnership throws up issues from earlier phases in the life cycle, offering both a requirement and an opportunity for reworking. It is usually the case that those couples presenting for marital therapy have not been able to manage that transition in some way or another, but they have covered up the difficulty with a defensive makeshift. Some work on their unresolved infantile conflicts is usually necessary to enable them to commit themselves more fully to an intimate relationship, but couples also have to live comfortably with what is *not* changed in each other, or, to put it more precisely, the dissatisfactions as well as the fulfilments have to be containable.

The greater the deprivation, the more difficult it will be to give up the omnipotent hope that a perfect marriage will compensate for the inadequacies of past relationships. The implicit longing for wholeness that fuels unconscious choice of partner is indistinguishable from the urge that propels people into individual therapy, notwithstanding that the one is entered into in happiness and the other in misery. Both kinds of therapeutic institutions need to keep the longing alive, but both must ultimately deal with the impossibility of its fulfilment. However, while this realization eventually leads to the ending of therapy, it provides the stimulation for the continuance of marriage as a "life-long conversation".

Paradoxically, it is those couples who cannot bear to let go of the magical hopes that have been glimpsed in the first flush of romantic love who find themselves caught in the endless repetition of old hurts and failures. Both the Blakes and the Halls demonstrate that a successful marriage depends not so much on the resolution of dissatisfaction as on a more creative means of managing it within the relationship. Many marriages contain quite gross areas of pathology (lack of integration) because it is integrated into the overall relationship.

Evelyn Cleavely goes so far as to suggest that the defensive system itself can form a crucial aspect of the container. As she puts it,

> The marriage relationship itself provides a kind of "container" in which the internal conflicts of each can be externalized and made accessible in the interactive processes the couple develop between them, keeping alive the hoped-for resolution of these conflicts, but within a defensive system that guards against the intolerable fears they are expected to arouse. [Cleavely, chapter four, this volume]

The defensive system thus both makes possible and limits what can be achieved within the relationship. Since it is, itself, a reflection of the couple's intolerable fears, it implies that these fears are not resolved or transcended nor even entirely integrated, but neither do they have to be resolutely avoided. Holding is perhaps a better image for this than defence, since, like defence, it implies protection but does not have the connotation of avoidance. This is why couples like the Halls and the Blakes find that they can now talk about areas that, if not total no-go areas, were previously strewn with mines. Although the Halls communicated much more of their fears of destructiveness, guilt, and loss to us than they became directly aware of themselves, they had an *experience* with us of these dangerous areas being far less explosive than they had feared. This therefore opened up the areas within which it was possible for them to communicate. If, as Gregory Bateson (1973) has argued, messages constitute the relationship, it is obvious that an enlargement of the total communication network is experienced by the couple as an enhanced and therefore more satisfying relationship.

Finally, there is one more requirement of a container, which was discussed earlier under the heading of the analytic container. This is the need for boundaries. While Cleavely's notion of the protective–defensive system describes one kind of boundary, a safe space needs protection not only from what is feared inside but also from what is outside. The couple need a shared private space from which others are excluded. This may be represented by the image of the closed bedroom door. This describes a boundary to protect not only the inside from the outside but also the outside from the inside. Just as couples may appropriately export their difficulties into the therapeutic container, they may less appropriately attempt to export them into their relatives—especially their children. Many of the difficulties children suffer are the result of evacuation out of the marital relationship of what the couple are unable to contain. Sexual abuse of children is an obvious example (see also Zinner & Shapiro, 1972). And, just as Freud forbade his patients to "leak" information vital to the treatment to others (Freud, 1913c), so does the marital couple need to be able to trust that what is exposed within their shared intimacy is not leaked elsewhere. Given that this is yet another of those tensions that have to be struggled with, I sympathize with those spouses who complain that their partner talks too much about their relationship to friends or relatives. This constitutes a defensive strategy against the intimacy of the couple—the fear that the container will become, as Meltzer puts it, a claustrum (Meltzer, 1982).

In conclusion, I would like to spell out what I see as the links in a chain of ideas that runs from Bowlby to Bion. Attachment is the behavioural expression of an emotional and psychological need for what Winnicott describes as holding. The mother who securely holds her baby forms a container whose

boundaries protect him and enable him to discover and to isolate the safe space that is the true self. Whether this true self be
regarded as primary or as created out of experience, it needs to
be articulated within the mother–child interaction, and this
function of articulation is what Bion refers to as the container/
contained apparatus.

Although this formulation is probably an over-simplifica-
tion, it draws attention to the extraordinary range of functions
the marital relationship is called upon to play. A good marital
container will include all these elements in a way that perhaps
no other adult relationship can do, with the exception of the
special situation of psychotherapy. While psychotherapy allows
for the repair of internalized functions of holding and containment by allowing the patient to regress and freeing him from
the requirements of a reciprocal relationship, marriage fosters
the continuing development of these functions within a relationship where transferences do not have to be dissolved and
projections can continue to be made. It is unlikely that any
relationship would be of much value if the partners were so
separate and integrated that they no longer needed to project.
Like wholeness, this is an ideal-type state that does not exist in
reality, where internal worlds are in continual interplay with
the internal worlds of others via external relationships with
those others. In a good marriage, however, which acts as a
containing relationship, there is sufficient alpha function to
allow projections to be processed and made available for introjection. It is not one partner or the other who is doing this but
both partners together as a function of the relationship that
exists between them.

NOTE

I would like to express my appreciation to Stanley Ruszczynski, whose
trenchant criticisms (and editorial tenacity) required me to make of this
a much better chapter than it would otherwise have been.

PART THREE

THE COUPLE AND THE INDIVIDUAL

Within the marital relationship the self-realisation of each partner is achieved *through the other* by the steady reality testing of the partner against the phantasies derived and transferred from earlier relations.

Tom Main

. . . the interplay between separateness and union.

Donald Winnicott

"If only we were more separate, we could stay together."

Douglas Woodhouse

INTRODUCTION

A predictable and inevitable dynamic in every couple relationship is that of the tension between, on the one hand, the needs and wishes of the individuals and, on the other hand, the requirements of the partnership they aspire to. Some individual needs, of course, can be, or will be sought to be, met only in the context of the committed couple relationship. However, in any healthy relationship there will always be a tension that may be simply summarized as that between dependence and independence. This dynamic has its roots in the earliest psychosomatic relationship between the mother and infant and takes on a fresh dimension during the earliest oedipal struggles, particularly in relation to the inevitable tension for the infant between his dependence on the parental couple *as parents* and his necessary separateness from the parental couple as a *sexual couple.* It is further replayed and reworked during the storms of adolescence and continues to play a part in every personal relationship.

In "Individuation in Marriage" (chapter six), Alison Lyons and Janet Mattinson ask as their central question whether a person can be a fully committed partner in a relationship *and* at the same time develop his own wholeness and capacity for individuation. By individuation they mean a self-realization that includes psychological integration as a result of the extension of consciousness. In a different conceptual framework this may be referred to as a taking back of projections and so a move from a more unintegrated paranoid–schizoid personality organization to a more depressive one—in short, a move towards psychological maturity.

Using a detailed illustration of a couple in psychotherapy, the two authors argue not only that such individuation is possible, but that the committed couple relationship can be viewed as a particularly effective vehicle for such an integration and maturation. This is brought about by the containment function usually sought in the unconscious contract of the couple relationship (as discussed in part two).

Warren Colman continues with the same theme in chapter seven, "The Individual and the Couple". He reminds us that when we speak of "marriage", we are using the word not only in the sense of the social reality of a marital couple, but also symbolically to refer to an *internal* capacity for marriage or coupling. This capacity is the capacity to allow opposites and differences to come together. This coming together, however, is not for the purpose of necessarily removing difference—that is a rather unrealistic idea—but more to find ways of managing the various struggles that the vicissitudes of life will inevitably bring with them.

In other words, Warren Colman is referring to the individual having an internalized image of a parental couple engaged in healthy and creative intercourse. This internal object relationship allows that individual the possibility of engaging in a variety of life pursuits where psychological "linking" may be required, not least of which is that of the couple relationship. Warren Colman ends on a realistic note when he writes that the couple relationship does not offer a solution to the hazardous adventure of living. Rather, it may provide a necessary starting place from which some of those hazards may be confronted with vigour and hope.

His final sentence is worthy of repetition. He writes, "Marriage does not have to be the place where I can entirely be myself, but it can be the place where I discover some of the possibilities for becoming myself" (p. 141).

The establishment of the internal capacity for "marriage" or linking depends on the successful negotiation of the oedipal struggles. In chapter eight, "The Impenetrable Other: Ambivalence and the Oedipal Conflict in Work with

Couples", James Fisher focuses on the Oedipus complex as the central concept in psychoanalysis and psychoanalytic psychotherapy with couples. In this seminal essay, James Fisher follows the development of Freud's thinking about the Oedipus complex in detail and highlights that its central dilemma is that of ambivalence. The complete understanding of the oedipal drama needs to include an awareness that however much the young child may strive for an affectionate relationship with the parent of the opposite sex (the so-called "positive" oedipal relationship), this must be with some degree of ambivalence because it may be experienced as threatening another important affectional attachment—that is, that to the other parent (the so-called "negative" oedipal relationship). Such an understanding may well be properly representative of the *triangular* nature of the oedipal situation. Furthermore, the child also has to secure the capacity to relate to a parental *couple*, who, by definition of their sexual relationship and generational difference, exclude the child from an area of intimacy. This relationship, too, the child can only achieve with ambivalence—with love *and* hate (the hatred being for being excluded).

Any intimate relationship, therefore, however much sought and desired, will have within it some degree of ambivalence. The capacity to tolerate this ambivalence may be said to be the resolution of the oedipal dilemma and be seen as requisite for the ability subsequently to create healthy personal relationships. "The opposite to love is not hate. These two always co-exist so long as there is a live relationship. The opposite to love is indifference" (Dicks, 1967).

Inherent in the hope invested in the betrothal of marriage lies the possibility of disappointment and ultimately betrayal. In her chapter, "Betrayal of Troth" (chapter nine), Janet Mattinson emphasizes that the experience of trust has within it the possible experience of betrayal. Betrayal can only come out of having trusted. We are not betrayed by our enemies, she says; it is our loved one who will hurt us and let us down. Using references primarily from literature and mythology, Janet Mattinson writes of the universality of the image of betrayal, be it in the biblical Judas, Shakespeare's Brutus, or in much contemporary literature.

What constitutes betrayal to any particular couple relationship depends on the conscious and unconscious covenant first made between them. The unfaithfulness that may be the cause of the sense of betrayal need not necessarily be only, or even primarily, a sexual unfaithfulness. The ordinary events of the possible and inevitable transitions of a couple's life—the birth of a child, adolescence, children leaving home, mid-life, ageing, and death—may be experienced, consciously or unconsciously, as a loss of the previously trusted and assumed—a betrayal. Whether such ordinary life events *are* experienced as a betrayal or managed as painful but developmental transitions depends on how developmental life events were contained for and by the infant and the child from the very beginning.

In the course of the ordinary psychological development of the infant, the disillusionment invited by the weaning mother, the realistic resolution of the Oedipus complex, and the withdrawal of projections in the move towards the depressive position may all be resisted as painful experiences of rejection and betrayal. Each, however, actually represents a step towards a psychological integration and maturation: a movement from omnipotence towards reality, a differentiation between self and other, and, ultimately, as discussed earlier, towards the toleration of ambivalence.

However, some experiences, be they for the infant, the child, or the adult, will be pathogenic and destructive—trust *will* have been betrayed. Janet Mattinson suggests that if forgiveness is not possible, revenge and cynicism may emerge as alternative responses. Future relationships will be undermined and attacked by cynical disbelief or the seeking for revenge.

Inherent, therefore, in the tension between the partners to a relationship, in terms of their individual aspirations and the opportunities and constraints offered by the other and by the relationship, lies the possibility for development and growth, with all the conflict and pain that this may appropriately involve. As psychotherapists, we are likely to be used by our patients to enable them to discover whether their conflict is one that is inherent in the development of the capacity for healthy and necessary ambivalence, or whether it is based on a betrayal that fundamentally and irrevocably destroys the basic trust required of any ongoing couple relationship.

CHAPTER SIX

Individuation in marriage

Alison Lyons and Janet Mattinson

I ndividuation *in* marriage? This title immediately raises the question of whether a person can partner another and, at the same time, develop his own wholeness and capacity for individuation. Or does he have to give up some of his drive towards wholeness in creating a viable partnership? Do the two aims conflict? Yes, at one level they do but, in doing so, they express a principle that runs through the writings of Jung. This is "the principle of opposition".

> A psychological theory, if it is to be more than a technical makeshift, must base itself on the principle of opposition; for without this it could only re-establish a neurotically unbalanced psyche. There is no balance, no system of self-regulation, without opposition. The psyche is just such a self-regulating system. [Jung, 1917]

In this chapter we illustrate this principle of opposition mainly through three interviews we had with a young couple who were in trouble with their marriage to the extent of believing that, although they did not want to, they might have to separate, such was the degree of frustration they were experiencing together. On their own they felt "stuck" and applied to the Tavistock Institute of Marital Studies for help.

Before describing this couple, their problem, and how they presented it to us, we define the terms in our title and the opposition inherent in them.

Individuation

We use Jung's definitions, of which there are several. In different contexts he varied the emphasis. "Individuation", he wrote in 1929, "means becoming a single, homogeneous being, and, insofar as 'individuality' embraces our innermost, last, and incomparable uniqueness, it also implies becoming one's own self. We could therefore translate individuation as 'coming to selfhood' or 'self-realisation'" (Jung, 1929). Later, he wrote, "I use the term 'individuation' to denote a process by which a person becomes a psychological 'in-dividual' (with a hyphen between the 'in' and the 'dividual'), that is, a separate indivisible unity or 'whole'" (Jung, 1934).

It is important to distinguish, as Jung did, between individuation and individualism (or egotism). Individualism means "deliberately stressing and giving prominence to some supposed peculiarities"; individuation is "the better and more complete fulfilment of the collective qualities of the human being". The idiosyncrasy of an individual therefore needs to be understood as the "unique combination, or gradual differentiation, of functions and faculties that in themselves are universal". Individuation is the expression of the collective by a unique individual. It aims at a "living co-operation of all factors". "The aim of individuation is nothing less than to divest the self of the false wrappings of the persona on the one hand and of the suggestive power of primordial images on the other" (Jung, 1934a).

It is, therefore, a process of maturation and, to use one of Jung's other definitions, a "search for the whole man".

The mind of the "whole man", however, consists of an unconscious as well as a conscious, and we, therefore, with Jung, have to add to our definitions of the process of individuation the integration of the conscious and unconscious. Progressive mental development requires an extension of consciousness.

When the individuation process was defined by Jung as a search for wholeness, it also became identified with religious or spiritual development, and Jung assumed that people would have time for this only in the second half of their lives, after they had established themselves in the world. Nevertheless, he also held the view that individuation is a *natural* process of maturation. He talked of the difference between someone being dragged (unconsciously) along the road to becoming an individual—towards their own full development—as compared with the person choosing (consciously) to walk this path upright. In his autobiography he showed that he knew a great deal about the distortions in human development that could be caused in childhood by disturbed parents and obtuse teachers, and the ensuing hindrance to individuation. Although he acknowledged that the natural process of maturation (laid down in the germ plasma) does not always go forward smoothly to fulfilment, any more than an acorn becomes an oak in the wrong climate, he was referring to the faulty climate of civilization. He did not concern himself with the detail of early developmental processes, to which latter-day Jungians, particularly in the London school, have addressed themselves. However, in this chapter we are referring to the concept of individuation in the first as well as the second half of life.

Howell, in speaking of that part of the individuation process which consists in recognizing and assimilating the shadow, described individuation as a "bitty job" that is started quite early in life (Howell, 1979). Zinkin, speaking of the process as observed in adolescence, said that adolescent "acting-out" and "dropping-out" should not be taken simply as a sign of "disturbance", since they contain attempts to develop and *become an individual* (Zinkin, 1979). He emphasized the idea that runs like a thread through all of Jung's writings, that regression to an undifferentiated state is not to be seen as purely negative: regression may enable the psyche to go forward in a new way. Individuation can occur at any crisis point in the life of an individual.

Marriage

In ordinary everyday terms, marriage can be defined as a committed, intimate partnership. This commitment is full of paradox. It offers a unique combination of the opportunity to regress within the intimacy of an on-going sexual relationship with, at the same time, the added responsibilities and ties of family life. We think of the ease with which adolescents turn from young adults into children and back again, and of the ease with which newly married but ordinarily well-controlled people can suddenly find to their dismay that they have started throwing plates at each other, and as suddenly can pull themselves together and go and greet their dinner guests. They are surprised to find that the physical freedom they can now enjoy together takes this unexpected turn and has been used to express anger as well as love.

Jung described marriage as an emotional "container" (Jung, 1925). This containment can be thought of in three ways: (1) The marriage itself is a container: in terms of a legal commitment, it is still more difficult and more costly to get out of than to get into. (2) One partner can contain the other partner. (3) One partner can be contained by the other.

Just as a young child needs to be contained, to be given a safe place or "breathing space" in which to be, and offered safety and security as a base from which to explore and develop his mastery of skills and to which to retreat when his efforts fail, so, too, might an adult develop more of his own fullness of nature if provided with an emotional container.

Some marriages are apparently based on one partner seeking containment, the other wishing and being able to provide this containment. Jung described the contained partner as feeling himself living wholly within the confines of his marriage. Outside he has few obligations or binding interests. A simpler nature, he said, works on a more complicated one like a room that is too small, not allowing the partner enough space. On the other hand, the more obviously complex partner gives the simpler nature of the other person too much space, so that he does not know where he belongs. The more complicated, who have a tendency to dissociate and "split off", have, perhaps, an even greater need to be contained, but then find that they cannot be absorbed, they feel increasingly outside the marriage, and they start, in his words, "spying out of the window". The more the contained clings, the more the container feels shut out. The more the contained pushes in, the less the container can respond, and, therefore, he provides confirmation of the insecurity that feels so painful to the one who asks to be contained.

Although some marriages appear to be based on one partner seeking containment and the other providing this, we believe from our experience of working with marital problems in the Tavistock Institute of Marital Studies that the obvious and conscious container is sometimes the unconsciously contained and, vice versa, the obviously and consciously contained is unconsciously and emotionally the container.

As an example, we think of Irene and Soames in *The Forsyth Saga*. Irene, on the face of it, had a much more complicated nature than Soames, she felt restricted and confined by him and increasingly outside the marriage. She then started "spying out of the window" at the more complex-seeming Bosiny. The more Soames pushed, the more she felt alienated, and the more he felt rejected, culminating in the famous so-called rape. Yet it was clear, after Irene left home, that she was badly in need of a container, and she finally found one in Jolyon.

In their marriage, both Irene and Soames maintained their positions as "strong-container" Irene and "weak-contained" Soames only by a very one-sided arrangement, which ignored parts of their own being. She was not aware of her emotional weakness, and he was not aware of his emotional strength, which, perhaps, they could discover only through their second marriages.

Marriage partners are in the greatest difficulty when both are desperately seeking to be contained and when such is the pressure of this need that they cannot start to perceive or recognize the equivalent need in the other and provide accordingly. They then become enmeshed in the desperate struggle of "who is to be the baby".

Opposition

In these definitions of individuation and marriage we have mentioned several pairs of opposites:

- the individual and the collective
- conscious and unconscious
- whole and part
- single person and partnership
- container and contained
- retreat and exploration
- looking in and looking out

In thinking about pairs of opposites, it is easy to think of one's self caught in a clinch of "either/or"—one or the other—and forget the space in-between. Remembering the definition of the psyche as a self-regulating system, the task of maturation is concerned with being able to stand in this space between the opposites and able to maintain the tension of opposing forces to an increasing degree. To give an example: imagine a child torn between the wish to keep the bag of sweets all for himself and the wish to please his mother's watchful eye and offer half to a young visitor. If the mother does not know about the tension of opposites in herself, she gives one of two polarized responses. Either she orders the child to behave nicely, or she leaves the child to handle the conflict on his own. The ordinary "good-enough" mother, able to hold tension within herself and maintain a position between these opposing standards, conveys to the child that his conflict is understood and that she herself knows about it, perhaps by saying something to the effect of "I think you can manage it".

Mr and Mrs Turner

Mr and Mrs Turner were a young couple who applied to the Institute for help with their marriage. We will describe the conflict they were experiencing in their attempts at individuation and in their attempts to be contained and to

contain each other. We can say that in their expressed
wish to stay married they were aware of their need to be
contained, despite the inherent conflict between their
complexity and simplicity, the need to "push in" and the
"spying out of the window".

They were both in their late twenties, and they had two
children, a little girl aged three and a little boy aged one.
Mr Turner worked as a greengrocer in a small but
expanding family business.

In making their application, they both wrote a letter. Mrs
Turner began by itemizing the problem:

1. too little sex (once a month);
2. too little communication;
3. too little sharing;
4. too little honesty;
5. too little trust;
6. I've tried too much of the time;
7. I don't want my husband in the sexual sense;
8. I haven't any interests;
9. I fear the loss of my identity, sense of belonging to
    this world, feeling of being important;
10. our two young children get me down;
11. my husband works long hours.

This list was followed by three pages of elaboration,
particularly regarding her husband's football, his dogs, his
time off, her pregnancies, and ending, "it sounds as if I
blame him for the agony of that pregnancy. I probably do,
but I don't think I'm still holding it over his head. . . . I get
confused trying to see the cause of our unhappiness."

Mr Turner's exposition of their problem was, on the face of
it, more vague and much less clearly set out than his
wife's, but on closer inspection the contents turned out to
be quite as strongly expressed as that of Mrs Turner.
Nevertheless, he ended with what turned out to be a
characteristic apology for "this rather confused

assessment of the situation". He did not itemize, but we extracted the important sentences and found we had a list consisting again of 11 items:

1. We are both unhappy.
2. Laura gets depressed and has no time for herself.
3. We find it difficult to communicate and often distrust each others' motives.
4. I find it difficult to manage the demands of being a husband and father and running a small family business.
5. I seem to be pressurized from both sides and crushed from both sides. This leads to frustration.
6. I get short-tempered.
7. I no longer have time for my hobbies.
8. Our sex life is non-existent.
9. I understand the reasons but still feel frustrated.
10. Laura has always said we have never repaired the damage done when we were first married (my time spent at the business and on hobbies), although at the time it didn't seem to be doing any damage.
11. I know there are many symptoms of our not making our marriage work, but I think we would both like it to.

We arranged to see Mr and Mrs Turner for a consultation, first on their own in single interviews and then the following week in a joint one.

MRS TURNER'S SINGLE INTERVIEW

Mrs Turner was a tall, slim, pretty girl, slightly childlike in face and bearing. On the day of her interview she wore an attractive velvet pinafore dress. Her long hair was taken back from her face, and her general appearance was of an old-fashioned teenager. If she had looked happier, one could have imagined her running around playfully, but she was too listless and depressed to run anywhere.

She made a considerable appeal. She was immediately tearful, perhaps by these tears trying to evoke help. Despite her tears and despite her complaining of difficulties in communicating with her husband and many times saying, "Perhaps I am not clear", her account and description of feelings were lucid.

The effect Mrs Turner had on her therapist was to make her work very hard. The therapist responded to Mrs Turner's appeal, and at the end of the interview felt most understanding. In retrospect she thought that she had been too helpful.

Mrs Turner described her problem in terms of her frustration in not being able to get her husband to be more at home, in not being able to get a response from him, of her tiredness, and of her very real fear that she might break down. Her frustration was the keynote in every situation she described. However, she felt guilty that her frustrated behaviour had got to a point of flinging objects around the house and screaming. She thought she had already harmed the children, and she was still petrified that she might "batter" the baby girl. We thought that her fear of what she might do to this child and the age of that child was related to her getting herself referred at this particular time.

She described the history of their marriage. They had met when she was in the first year of her job as a librarian. She went out on a blind date with him, and after three more outings felt she might marry him because she felt "good with him". Looking back, however, she thought they never could communicate—they were "poles apart" and saw things "very differently". She described herself as being introspective. She used to read a lot and, except when in wild frustration, she studied her behaviour and what she should say and what she should not say.

Before the birth of the first baby, sex, to her, felt good. Since then she felt that her husband "only used" her. She

was mainly too tired for sex, so they seldom had it; then it
was "all right".

As regards her personal history, she told the therapist that
she was the younger of two girls. Her father had been in
the Army during and after the war. This meant a lot of
moving around and her going to several different primary
schools. On these family postings she remembered bitter
quarrels between her parents. She also remembered her
mother speaking bitterly of her resentment at having been
left on her own with two babies on earlier unaccompanied
postings. Her mother despised her father's social status
and his choice of job when he came out of the Army. Her
father expected excessively high standards from her in
things like deportment, table manners, and school
performance, which she and her sister could never attain.
Her parents' quarrels were often about these aspirations,
so that she felt herself to be the object of the quarrel. Her
mother did not expect nearly so much from her. In fact, it
sounds as if she expected too little. When Mrs Turner
wanted help with something, her mother did not encourage
and assist her but took over the job and did it for her.

Outside school Mrs Turner had few interests, and when
she was a teenager she spent much of her time asleep.
This made the therapist wonder if she had been very
depressed at that age, although she did well enough at
school to get herself to University. When she first started
working, she found the job a very great strain, as her
expectations of herself were so high—she wanted to be the
librarian of all children's librarians. She was extremely
critical of parents when they slapped their children for
minor misdemeanours in the library.

Mr Turner's single interview

The immediate impression that Mr Turner gave was of a
"country boy". He had a freshly complexioned face and
short hair. He wore a leather jacket and a home-knitted

sweater. He could have been a stable lad or a young farmer. At the beginning of the session he was fairly tongue-tied but was not unduly embarrassed by this.

When he spoke of their problem, he described a confused malaise (not his word). Things were not very bad, but they were certainly not right. He could not blame himself or his wife—he was just bewildered.

Before he met and married Mrs Turner, he had had several girlfriends, but never more than one at a time, and he had always been very serious about them and found he easily got involved. His friends used to tease him that he should take things more lightly. He also described the blind date on which he and Mrs Turner had met. He said that he had been attracted to her for her lively mind and because she was different from any of his previous girlfriends and from himself.

It became increasingly clear through the interview that he experienced the world through his senses, particularly through touch, and now he felt very rejected *physically*, not just sexually, by his wife. Contrary to what Mrs Turner said, he described sex as always having been disappointing. He still found her very attractive sexually, but he had to "manage without" and felt very deprived by this. He seemed to have a great need to touch and be touched, and the therapist began to think that he might be taking unconscious revenge for the sexual deprivation by absenting himself emotionally from his wife.

However, he seemed to be trying quite consciously not to over-compensate for the rejection by his wife by making it up with the children. He was very aware that his wife had to put up with them all day, and he was a novelty when he came home. He described an incident of the previous evening, when the little girl had refused to kiss her mother good-night when he was going to put them to bed. He could see how hurt his wife had been, and he insisted after they got upstairs that the child went back and kissed her mother. He seemed very identified with his wife over this incident, and, as we talked, he began to realize how his being so absorbed in the television when she wanted to talk, and playing football most of his free time, were ways of getting his own back, although he said he had not thought of this before.

He was the eldest of four children. His parents came from an impoverished background and were still poor when he was a small child. His parents started their married life in one room in the grandparent's home and did not move until after the second child was born. He always felt his father preferred the next boy and that his mother preferred the third. But his mother would stand up for him against his father if necessary. Although he did not like his father, he remembered with pleasure occasions when they all went out collecting wood together; he talked nostalgically about forests, dogs, and gravel pits.

When he left school, he tried a job in a factory, disliked it, and then went to work with his father in the greengrocery business. Working hard, they had prospered, and he could understand why his mother, who had had a very deprived and poor childhood, being one of thirteen, now "threw" the money around. This shocked his wife very much and was quite at odds with her middle-class standards.

He and his brother had now taken over the management of the business from their father, and although he found this a worry, he clearly also enjoyed the work. He was very keen on his dogs and trained them regularly in his lunch hour. He became quite authoritative when he gave a detailed explanation of how "dogs learnt by association". Then he stopped himself, saying that it must seem as if he were more interested in dogs than in children, but really that was not so. He felt sad that his wife did not share any of his enthusiasms and could not understand, for instance, that he preferred to work out things for himself. She got upset when he refused to read "the Directions".

The therapist thought she could hear the disappointed undertones of the small boy whose mother had not had time to play with him and enjoy him, and in whose childhood dogs had probably supplied the most unconditional admiration and love. But his reflective manner, his interested and undefensive acceptance of the link between his feelings of rejection and the way he absented himself from situations, made her feel hopeful about the prospect of working with him. He was likeable and with apparently no idea that this was so.

JOINT INTERVIEW WITH MR AND MRS TURNER

He and Mrs Turner chose to sit side by side in this interview. Mrs Turner opened it and remarked that her single interview had been meaningful to her in terms of "not being misunderstood". It was interesting that she put it this way round and did not say that she felt "understood". The importance was in *not being misunderstood*. Then she started to question the two therapists in a searching way as to what they had thought of her and her husband. Behind her actual words the big question seemed to be, "Do you value us, will we do, was I a good enough client?" She put the expectations of good behaviour onto the therapists. Mr Turner wanted to talk more about their problem of communication and the conversation he had had in his previous interview about their not believing that the other's means of conveying information—hers verbal, his physical—was communicating. He said he had been very nervous about the single interview but had found it easier than he had expected; but now he was nervous of the joint one. The therapists learnt that, on their way home together, the couple, who had had their individual interviews at the same time, had been able to discuss their individual experiences. After that they had obviously avoided talking about the problem; business had taken up his time, and their mutual tiredness in the evenings had prohibited further communications, either verbal or physical, between them. It seemed that they had left the two interviews with renewed hope, but they had not been able to translate this into any action, and both had retreated into work, tiredness, and sleep.

Then, in a circular way, they re-stated their problem. Mrs Turner expressed it in terms of loss of respect for each other, never having been able to discuss anything, even when engaged, and now being more stuck than ever, leaving a void and emptiness between them. Mr Turner kept on emphasizing what he had understood about their different ways of communicating. None of the comments the therapists made shifted their circular conversation. They went round the circle again, until she started to cry and then apologized profusely for crying. He could not comfort her. The therapists commented on the crying as a communication. This astounded Mr Turner, who said that he had "never thought of that". He said he would have comforted her at home but was too embarrassed to do it in the clinic.

Then Mrs Turner became quietly accusing of the time Mr Turner spent at the business, on his hobbies, and with his dogs. He quietly stood up for himself and insisted that a lot of what she complained about was in the past, not in the present. His hurt about her physical rejection of him showed through, although he had physically rejected her tears. She became more angry as he became more hurt, and she became particularly angry that he was not getting angry at her, feeling that she was not getting a response but, in fact, not noticing his hurt.

She exhibited clearly how she nagged at him and went on and on trying to get the response she wanted. At one point he corrected her and then pointed out to the therapists that his voice had risen and he had been made very angry by her remarks. "You've seen I'm cross, haven't you?" he asked. It had been just barely visible to a carefully watching eye.

She accused him of loving his dogs more than the children. He denied this and said that he trained his dogs only in his lunch hour. At this stage of the interview, they sounded as if they were "auctioneering". She said, "you

did" so and so, and he said, "I didn't do" so and so, "I did"
such and such. She modified the so and so, he modified
the such and such, the argument had a rising crescendo,
and then the hammer came down on some agreement.
They repeated the auctioneering on several points at issue.

In standing up for himself, Mr Turner emphasized his
concern for the future and bettering the business, so that
he could give her and the children more security. He
seemed to be more related to the future, she to his past
misdeeds. The auctioneering seemed some attempt to get
things a bit more into the present.

At the end, Mrs Turner said the joint interview had been
helpful because she could not get hysterical, and Mr
Turner could not leave and go into the kitchen. Apparently
the therapists had provided some containment.

A fee and possible times for future appointments then had
to be negotiated. At her previous single interview Mrs
Turner had made some difficulty about the timing of the
joint appointment, saying she could manage any day, but
she doubted whether her husband could get out of the
business. In this final negotiation, he was quite clear that
he could manage any afternoon and that he was prepared
to pay as much as he could afford and even cut down on
some other expenditure to enable them to come. It was
very clear that she did not notice that he was prepared to
make this effort and find the money.

Discussion

In discussing this material, we come back to the principle of
opposition as expressed in the inherent conflict between the
process of individuation and the process of sharing in marriage—or, as we might say, who within a marriage contains
whom.

In doing this, we look at the interview material under three
headings: (1) the courtship and choice of partner; (2) the on-
going difficulties within the marriage; and (3) something of

what we believed this couple would need to work at together in their therapy.

Choice of partner

In their choice of partner, Mr and Mrs Turner consciously chose a person similar to themselves in one main respect. They both consciously rejected the model of marriage offered to them by their parents. Mrs Turner did this explicitly and said, with enormous emphasis, that she did not want her marriage to be like that of her parents. They both chose a partner who was seemingly very different from their parent of the opposite sex.

However, they also chose a partner who was complementary to themselves. Mr Turner had grown up in a situation where, by necessity, physical survival of the family group was all-important. Individuals did not get much noticed, and he chose a partner who represented more culture, more words, more education—"her lively mind," as he said. Mrs Turner chose a partner who represented fewer words, the less educated, the more earthy and practical.

In Jung's terms, they chose a partner who exhibited and used the mental function they themselves used least. He distinguished four functions—those of sensation, intuition, thinking, and feeling, the first two of these relating to perception, the second two to the ordering of the perception (Jung, 1921). From the limited knowledge of Mr and Mrs Turner acquired in two interviews, the therapists guessed that the function Mr Turner used most was that of sensation, but that he appeared to have difficulty in ordering and knowing about these perceptions and wanted Mrs Turner to do this for him. Mrs Turner seemed to be a feeling type, which enabled her to arrive at a value judgement without using a conscious logical process. As she said, "I wanted to marry him because I felt good; I can't explain it further".

She may well have meant by this that she felt more able to be herself when with him and in these terms was seeking an opportunity for and containment in which to individuate and walk more upright.

Her model of masculinity, husbanding, and fathering had been one of high expectations, which left her defeated and never able to attain to the good behaviour that was demanded of her. She chose a husband who had fewer words with which to tell her what to do. His expectations were there in the background, but were expressed in his work and in developing a business. Consciously she had chosen a man who was the opposite of her father; unconsciously she had chosen a man also with high ideals as regards their future security.

Mr Turner's model of femininity had been one of a work-ridden life and with little time to notice his difference and individuality. With little noticing going on around him, he developed his own noticing (or perceiving), and he married a girl who seemed to notice him quickly and who, socially and culturally, had time to notice. In actual fact, her noticing was very limited.

They chose, on her instigation, to live in an isolated cottage, where, no doubt, as she thought, she would be able "to be herself", not demanded of by relatives, friends, and neighbours; he raised no objection, and probably this idea met his wanting to be the only person around whom she could notice.

The difficulties in the on-going marriage

Mr and Mrs Turner were immediately in difficulties in their marriage and unconsciously defeated their conscious intentions, little noticing how, in rejecting certain hated characteristics in their parents, they, at the same time, re-employed these modes of behaviour.

Mrs Turner, just as she had intended to be the best librarian of all children's librarians, tried to have the perfect marriage, be the wife of all wives, and the mother of all mothers. She imposed her own demands, instead of those of her father, on herself and on her husband; perhaps she was trying to get Mr Turner to feel like what she herself had experienced all her life.

More overtly complex than he and more obviously the container, she frantically sought containment and then failed to notice him and his need to be contained. The more she pushed, the more he "spied out of the window" into the business. As she said, in response to her pleas and hysterics, he had reduced his working hours and had taken his turn in getting up to the children at night, but always it was felt by her not to be enough and always too late: what she was getting now, she needed then. In the joint interview, it took a three-minute auction for her to concede the point that he did, in fact, now do what she accused him of not doing.

Mr Turner, in his search for his whole self, particularly his masculinity, although apparently a simpler character, found not enough room for his development within the confines of her demands. He was only noticed as an extension of herself; the more she tried to push into him, the more he retreated into his work and his football. He found comfort with his dogs, who valued his hands rather than deriding them. He sought further definition of himself outside the marriage and, in doing this, he contained her less and therefore increased her insecurity.

They soon ceased to value each other's major mental function. She could not bear it when he worked things out with his hands and refused to read the directions on the box. Her words became more hysterical and less meaningful to them both. The part of themselves they denied and could not use, which they needed the other to express for them, became despised.

They could not, as they said, communicate. We believe that one of their difficulties in this was that in attempting to better and correct the past, Mrs Turner was stuck in it; Mr Turner, in attempting to better and realize himself, was as defensively ignoring the present and projecting his expectation and idealization into the future.

IN CONCLUSION

Finally, we come back to the principle of oppositions, and, in doing so, we implicitly state what we believe is the emotional task of marriage—any marriage—and what we believed would be the task of the therapy with this couple, who had stated their wish to remain married.

Remembering the definitions of individuation we used and the ordinary everyday definition of marriage as a partnership, we again ask, can a person partner another at the same time as developing his wholeness and his own capacity for walking upright? We believe not only that he can, but that, in using Jung's definition of marriage as the container, the marriage can be used as a vehicle for maturation and for becoming a more complete person.

In saying that marriage can be used as a container in which people can develop their own wholeness, we are not saying that it is necessarily used by everyone, nor that it is the only possible container for this task. We are, however, saying that it is a particularly useful container because, by its structure, it keeps the individual in intimate touch with another as well as himself. As Jung said,

> Individuation has two principal aspects; in the first place it is an internal and subjective process of integration, and in the second it is an equally indispensable process of objective relationship. Neither can exist without the other, although sometimes the one, and sometimes the other predominates. [Jung, 1934a]

Looking around at people's marriages, both as they exhibit them to their friends and relatives and as they describe and enact their marital relationship in the presence of a therapist, it seems that marriages in our Western culture can be divided into two types (with, of course, various shadings in-between). There are those couples who enter marriage with the express purpose of providing themselves with a container in which the expression of instinctual drive, feeling, and conflict is avoided; this is a totally defensive manoeuvre. And there are those who enter marriage with either the conscious or the unconscious purpose of finding a container that will give them room in which to be, and for the expression of instinctual drives and feelings, so that they may further their development and come to know more fully the different parts of themselves, eventually getting these parts into a more satisfying conjunction; this in itself will raise tension of one sort or another, both internally and between the partners, though not necessarily the type of auction and hysterics displayed by Mr and Mrs Turner.

We wish to stress that we do not believe that conflict in itself is a negative factor. Obviously it can be expressed in a disturbing, destructive, and rejecting way, as the Turners were experiencing. But it can also be the means of growth, and we suggest that it offers more potential for growth than a strict adherence to a principle of avoidance of conflict and opposition, inculcating, as this does, so much defensive denial of the unintegrated reality and fullness of the self.

Mr and Mrs Turner married each other on a very hopeful basis of finding someone who expressed unrealized parts of themselves with which they wanted to identify—or, as we may say, with which they wanted to keep in touch. Mrs Turner was quite explicit that her choice was based on wanting to be able to be more herself and seeing Mr Turner as a means of doing this.

Their immediate expression of their difficulties was also hopeful in that they felt safe enough to test out their difficulties and to try and find a corrective experience with each other. The containment of marriage allows for some regression, and, if worst fears are not realized, there is the chance to go forward again.

Mr and Mrs Turner were in continued and increasing trouble when they felt their deepest fears of being rejected were realized—a rejection of what they were trying to become, as opposed to what they had always been expected to be. For Mr Turner this was mainly a physical experience. For Mrs Turner it was mainly an emotional experience, and it may be that it was because she was so out of touch with her body that her feelings rose to such an hysterical level. Bodies are good anchors of feelings.

Although Mr and Mrs Turner were consciously anxious to do better for themselves and for their children than they felt their own parents had done for them, such was the strength of the unconscious attachment to these parents that they found themselves repeating a familiar pattern. As much as Mrs Turner consciously despised her parents and as much as Mr Turner felt he had not had enough from his, neither of them had the capacity to relinquish that anger, because, as unindividuated as they were with not enough emotional autonomy, they had not acquired the capacity to discriminate between past and present, and between future and present.

Mrs Turner, for example, was still ruled by an internalized demand to be perfect. It is difficult to imagine from her description of her childhood that Mrs Turner's father ever said, "I think you can manage it". He just told her what she ought to be, leaving her a failure. Mr Turner was left to find himself, but he also had no one to say, "You can do this," or even notice that he wanted to do it. Without any fundamental belief that they could do it, they easily gave up and slipped back into an old familiar pattern of behaviour. She started despising him, as she had despised her parents. He retreated from her and got himself unnoticed, as he had been unnoticed in the past. He, disappointed by the lack of containment she gave him, immediately retreated to his work, his sport, his dogs, and the far-distant future. She then became more and more frustrated and more and more hysterical in her chase of him.

Both of them, like most people, brought many infantile needs, which had not been met earlier in their lives, into the marriage. Such, however, was the urgency of the drive for containment of this couple that they failed to notice the need and "the child" in the other.

We believe that the process of individuation should not be thought of only as a process of linear development and as an attempt to leave "the child", which lives in us all, behind. As Jung said, the attempt to leave "the child" behind denies a part of ourselves and results in unconscious behaviour of a very childish, as opposed to childlike, behaviour. A more conscious recognition of the childlike in ourselves and in other people, and providing containment for this for ourselves and for others so that it can be brought into a happier and less destructive balance with the more adult components of our personalities, is more upright than dragging the unconscious child behind.

Parents seem to relate better to their children if they can remain in touch with childlike aspects of their own personalities; and they are more able to help their children develop more fully if they themselves are in the process of bringing their own living child into better conjunction with their adult self.

Mr and Mrs Turner had "lost respect" for each other and had come to despise in the other the rejected parts of themselves. As Jung said, many people remain deliberately unconscious about much of their behaviour in an attempt to avoid

conflict within themselves and knowing about their own ambivalence. If the conflict cannot be contained and tolerated
within the person, it becomes externalized into the relationship, and one half of the split is projected into the partner.

In these terms, the therapy with Mr and Mrs Turner needed
to be concerned with their starting to provide a mutual containment that would feel safe enough for them to dare to discover
the parts of themselves they had rejected. Only then would they
be able to move forward on the path towards individuation.
Knowing more about these parts in themselves, they would be
more likely to be, not only more upright, but also less despising, and more valuing of these attributes in the other. Or, in
other words, we could say the therapy would be about helping
them to extend their level of consciousness and become more
aware of some of their at present unconsciously formed behaviour.

Remembering Mr Turner's plea in the joint interview, "Did
you notice that I was angry?" we can state the therapeutic task
in their terms:

- to help them notice themselves more;
- to help Mrs Turner to notice Mr Turner more;
- to help Mr Turner to trust in and order his perceptions more.

Or finally, in Jung's terms, we could say that the therapeutic
task would be to help them provide a more balanced and flexible container for each other, she less pushing in, he less
pushed into "spying out of the window", so that within the
togetherness they could continue to know themselves more
fully and continue in their life task, as human beings, of developing their wholeness, self-regulating the tension of opposites
within themselves and between each other.

CHAPTER SEVEN

The individual and the couple

Warren Colman

The notion of psychic development is central to psycho-dynamic thinking. In this chapter I want to discuss my understanding of what this idea means and to place marriage within it. Marriage can either promote or restrict psychic development, and this issue leads directly to the role of marital therapy in promoting a psychic attitude that I describe as the internal marriage.

I do not intend to give a definition of psychological health, as that would imply the existence of some hypothetical end-point to development, a stage at which someone might be said to have achieved whatever goal was thought to be desirable. There are a number of these in psychoanalytic currency, but they tend to be depressingly normative and rest on the resolution of particular developmental crises, such as the Oedipus complex or, in Melanie Klein's thinking, the depressive position. Freud's own dictum, that health involves the capacity to love and to work, has a terse universal ring of truth about it, but, even so, development is not so much an achievement as a goal—something that is not reached but is striven for. And unless we want to conscript everybody into our own mental health army, we have only to look around us to see how varied are the adaptations that individuals make to their lives and how creative some of the least normative of these are. Nor must we confuse health with an absence of suffering.

Development is something that goes on throughout life and includes the processes of ageing and decay, and ultimately death itself. Our understanding of it must be broad enough to include our going hence as well as our coming hither—it is something that encompasses the entire life-cycle. Life involves a continual process of adaptation, not only to the physical and psychological changes within ourselves, but also to the changes in the world around us. All of us have to negotiate the so-called psycho-social transitions involving our changing place and perspective in the life-cycle, and, in a period of rapid social change such as we now seem to be perpetually living through, there are much wider changes to negotiate as well. These changes require an attitude involving both flexibility and stability. As the hippies used to say twenty years ago, you have to "go with the flow". The same water flows into different places in the river and the same place on the river has a constant flow of different water. The river is stable, but the water is in constant movement. Only something that is stable can maintain itself in conditions requiring great change and adaptation, and, conversely, without flexibility stability becomes stubborn resistance, and when the pressure of change mounts it is likely to be swept away. These attributes of stability and flexibility have relevance both to social institutions, from nation states to individual marriages and families, and to the psychological institution of the self. One of the defining features of the self is thus continuity through change, though the exact nature of what it is that is continuous is as elusive—and as vitally important—as the Holy Grail. Development is more about what happens on the Quest than the finding of what is sought. While we may have intimations into the heart of the mystery, the Quest is a never-ending one.

The focus on the self as the touchstone of psychic development is a distinguishing feature of Jung's concept of individuation (Jung, 1934a). Individuation refers to the process of becoming an in-dividual—i.e. something both separate and unique and also whole and undivided. Jung describes it as a spontaneous, natural process by which a person becomes their own self, thereby realizing their potential. He compared it to what makes a tree grow into a tree: "if it is interfered with, then it becomes sick and cannot function as a tree, but left to itself it develops into a tree". But whatever wholeness or personal integration may be achieved, it is always relative: "the complete realisation of our whole being is an unattainable ideal. But unattainability is no argument against the ideal, for ideals are only signposts, never the goal" (McGuire & Hull, 1978).

Although individuation is a unique constellation in each individual, it is made up of the progressive differentiation of features that are themselves universal. Certain typical motifs, which Jung refers to as archetypes and which have correlations with Kleinian unconscious phantasies, occur again and again. This has immense importance for the stance we take towards the manifestations of shared unconscious phantasies in marriage. It suggests that they should not be regarded merely as an impediment to the relationship but, rather, as its basic substratum, even its driving force. The question, as with Jung's archetypes, is whether the marriage is in the grip of its phantasies, to the extent of being lived by them, or is able to act as a developmental vehicle for them. In the latter case, the marriage fosters the individuation of its participants and may even be said to have an individuation process of its own—after all, every marriage is different, just as every individual is different. Where individuation is occurring in an unimpeded way, conscious and unconscious operate in harmony, enabling the progressive differentation and integration of unconscious contents into a uniquely dynamic whole.

The process may be compared to the development of a piece of music, which, likewise, is basically made up of a remarkably small number of recurring elements. And, like the psyche, music is based on the principle of opposition, as a musician patient of mine pointed out to me recently. She had felt for some time that she and I were going in opposite directions. Whenever I made an interpretation, she sank into silence, feeling that my words were like enormous signposts forcing her to go in the direction I indicated because they obscured the much smaller, less defined signposts of her own inadequately formulated direction. But then she said, "that's the good thing about music—you can have two different things going on at the same time". And, I added, it's that which makes the music. The two things are also not necessarily in harmony—harmony includes the creative use of disharmony. This is a beautiful illustration of Jung's idea of the transcendent function of the psyche—its capacity to produce symbols that transcend the opposites and enable further development to take place (Jung, 1958). My patient and I have been more successful in making "music" together since this symbol emerged, and such transcendent symbols are an absolute necessity in the regulation of that archetypally warring pair of opposites, the married couple.

Marriage in development
and development in marriage

The principle of opposition—the idea that there is always a tension in the psyche between opposing forces—is fundamental to psychodynamic thinking. If the opposites can work together by means of the transcendent function, the tension between them becomes creative but is not dissolved. When the opposites are felt to be irreconcilable, splitting and polarization occur. Jung's idea of the psyche as a self-regulating system based on the balance of opposites is similar to the family systems notion of homeostasis, the way in which a family strives to achieve a workable balance between its opposing forces. This is another way of stating the developmental potential of marriage, since, if it is to be successful, it requires the capacity to sustain the tensions arising from a whole host of oppositions—e.g. my needs vs. your needs, separateness vs. togetherness, autonomy vs. dependence, love vs. hate, exploration vs. safety, similarity vs. difference, and, indeed, defence vs. development—the list is potentially endless. The title of this chapter describes one of the main parameters of these oppositions, the individual and the couple. This tension is well put by Lyons and Mattinson, who raise the question of whether "a person can partner another and, at the same time, develop his own wholeness and capacity for individuation. Or does he have to give up some of his drive towards wholeness in creating a viable partnership?" (chapter six, this volume).

As part of their answer, Lyons and Mattinson quote Jung, who states that individuation is not only "an internal and subjective process of integration", but also "an equally indispensable process of objective relationship. Neither can exist without the other" (Jung, 1946). Jolande Jacobi, addressing the same issue, says, "Excessive self-reliance makes for spiritual pride, sterile brooding, and isolation within one's own ego. Man needs an opposite to concretize his experience. Without the presence of someone other and different, question and answer merge into a formless mass" (Jacobi, 1942).

Nowadays we would see Jacobi's warning as relating to a description of narcissism, a pathological and defensive state resulting from early developmental failure in the establishment of a secure separate identity from which to relate to others. As the name implies, it is a disturbance of the sense of self. Such people feel themselves to be too fragile to risk involvement with others, and they defend themselves by withdrawing all their emotional investment into the narrow compass of self. Their dilemma is expressed by Hamlet's cry, "I could be bounded in a nutshell and count myself a king of infinite space were it not that I have bad dreams".

The individual self cannot develop in isolation. The I is defined by its differentiation from the You, and the You is required to provide an answer for the basic question of identity: Who am I? This question, although so fundamental, only becomes problematic when relationships with others are disturbed and unable to provide the necessary complement to self-realization. I am not, of course, suggesting that the I is only a function of what others take me to be—compliance with others in this way results in what Winnicott called the "false self" (Winnicott, 1960b). The true self, by contrast, can only flourish through interaction with others in which it receives affirmation and recognition that is congruent with its own experience—a process of validation that confirms the self as real.

Winnicott has described how this initially takes place in early infancy via the mother's mirroring of her baby. The baby looks at the mother's face and sees himself. As Winnicott puts it: "The mother is looking at the baby and what she looks like reflects what she sees there" (Winnicott, 1960a). This image indicates the power of the early mothering experience in the development of the individual. As Winnicott once said, there is no baby without a mother. At the beginning it is only possible to speak of the nursing couple (Winnicott, 1960a). Only later does the baby become a going concern in its own right, able to take on for itself some of the functions provided by the mother. The capacity for self-reflection, the *sine qua non* of human consciousness, is thus originally dependent on reflection by another.

However, to fulfil her mirroring function, the mother clearly must have the capacity for accurate empathy and responsiveness. She must be sufficiently merged with her infant to function as a part of itself—what Kohut calls a selfobject—but not so merged that she cannot distinguish between herself and the baby. In other words, she must herself have a clear and secure sense of self to be able to impart this to her baby. Otherwise the reflection will be distorted by her own narcissism—the tendency to treat the baby as though it is a part of herself. Babies are, unfortunately, excellent vehicles for projective identification, perhaps even better than spouses. Thus the baby may be regarded as an embodiment of the mother's own rage, greed, helplessness, damage, or whatever and treated accordingly. It is just as damaging to the baby to be neglected because the mother repudiates her own instinctual needs, as it is to be smothered because the mother attempts to use the baby to vicariously fulfil all that she feels is lacking in herself.

Although the roots of the individuation process are established early in life, it is, as I have said, a life-long process. Clearly, if the soil is poor, a tree will have the greatest difficulty realizing its full potential. There is more to a tree than its roots, however—it also has leaves, branches, and a crown. It needs sun and rain and an atmosphere free of toxic pollutants, and these needs continue throughout its life. Similarly, although the roots of individuation are in the early mother–infant interaction, the developing individual requires a facilitating environment throughout life. Even once we are established as separate individuals, we continue to need others to fulfil certain functions for us if we are to reach our full potential.

This is vividly illustrated by the mutual dependence of male and female in the act of sexual intercourse, with its inherent potential for the creation of new life. The mouth–nipple conjunction of the nursing couple is superseded by the penis–vagina conjunction of the copulating couple—a natural symbol for the union of opposites. Whatever one's view of the relativity of gender differences, the necessity of the other who is required to complete the self is powerfully symbolized by the complementarity of male and female. Despite the critique from the feminist lobby, in clinical practice I find that penis envy is surprisingly common in women, but then so, too, in men is fear of the vagina and envy of the woman's child-bearing capacity. These envious phenomena need be understood in terms of the narcissistic hatred of the dependency on others, needed for the fulfilment of self. The physical realities are inescapable and therefore make powerful symbolic images.

What I have been leading up to all this time can now be stated: marriage is not only a vehicle for development, it is itself a major requirement of the individuation process. But before objections are raised on behalf of the unmarried, let me explain that I am referring to marriage, and to the sexual act, as both a reality and a symbol. I am referring to the *internal capacity for marriage* or, to put it another way, the capacity to allow the opposites to come together inside the self in the inner world, in all the creative tension of an internal marriage. Real marriage both promotes and requires this capacity, and in this sense marital difficulties can be seen in terms of the couple's struggle to make an internal marriage. But, of course, there are many other ways of achieving the same aim—one thinks of the artist's relation to his work or the religious person's relation to God. But, in less obvious ways, any relationship with something or someone other that engages us on a deep level of our inner being and recognizes the reality of difference provides fruitful potential for working at the marriage of the opposites. Another way of putting this would be to describe it as the capacity for intimacy, since intimacy implies differentiation and separation: the sharing of our innermost being with another. Without separateness, intimacy becomes conflated with fusion: many couples cannot feel intimate unless they feel the same as their partner. Since this can rarely be the case, they are in a state of constant frustration and disappointment and tend to work harder and harder at trying to get the other to conform to their view of what they should be. In fact, because they cannot tolerate separateness, they cannot achieve intimacy either and are therefore condemned to the sterile coldness of isolation indicated in the previous quote from Jolande Jacobi. Separateness is felt to herald the catastrophe of complete abandonment and the attempt at fusion is thus a shared defence against acknowledging its reality.

Difficulties in the achievement of the internal couple

It should now be clear that I am proposing a psychological definition of marriage that is quite different from what is meant by legal marriage and even the looser definition that takes account of committed partnerships that have not been legally endorsed. According to this definition, a couple may have been legally married for a lifetime but never have achieved the psychological marriage of opposites. In fact, the psychological marriage is, like development itself, a life-long task, a *magnum opus*. But lest it be thought that I am speaking of some obscure esoteric procedure only practised by a few psychotherapeutic initiates, let me remind the reader that this definition is a commonplace. For surely it is what is meant when people say that marriage is something you have to work at. Yet few of us are prepared for what that really means: we prefer to go on in our old ways and are continually upended and discomforted by our partner's reminders that there is another to consider in all their irreducible difference.

A couple who came for an emergency consultation epitomized this discomfort in extreme form. For many years the wife had allowed herself to be virtually taken over by her husband. She had stayed at home looking after the children while he made all the decisions, not only about the home but even to the extent of buying her clothes for her. He complained that she would not do anything herself and therefore left him no choice. There was a heated argument about decorating the bedroom, which both of them saw as an example of their not being able to do anything together. It turned out that he had insisted it should be painted black. She could not make her protests heard and therefore saw no reason why she should co-operate in choosing carpets and curtains for this bedroom she did not want in the first place. Instead, she had decorated another room using delicate Laura Ashley prints (floral patterns and pastel colours). She gave this as evidence that she was more capable than he was making her out to be.

I was interested in the fact that, unusually, they had made a point of telling me about their backgrounds early on in the interview. They particularly wanted me to know that both sets of parents had divorced in their early childhoods. I could now see why they wanted me to know this. I pointed out to them their shared lack of an internal couple capable of remaining together through differences. Their various attempts at dealing with this difficulty had all resulted in failure. They had attempted the fusion of having one partner incorporated by the other. The wife felt stifled, and the husband felt overburdened. Then, over the issue of the bedroom, they had polarized: he went for an extreme stereotype of masculinity, she for one of femininity. Neither could engage in intercourse with the other, in any sense of the word. Psychologically as well as physically they were living in separate rooms, isolated not only from the frustrations but also from the satisfactions of sharing. Having failed to fuse and failed to split, they resorted to a third well-worn alternative—they began to fight. But this at least was closer to health, since it involved the recognition of an other who was different and opposed to themselves.

This too, though, can become an entrenched pattern—just as fusion can be used to avoid separateness, so can fighting be used to avoid togetherness. But the underlying difficulty is the same in both cases—there is no image of a genuine two-some, a couple. Instead, there are felt to be only the alternatives of a one-person fusion or a complete banishment to the outer darkness, ultimately annihilation. It came as no surprise to hear that this particular couple had had virtually no sex for several years and presented in a crisis at the point when the wife had had a brief affair. Suddenly the shared defence reversed, and instead of the wife being the helpless and dependent one, the husband was forced to acknowledge his enormous dependency on her. He was terrified that she would leave him.

Affairs like these frequently represent a bid for freedom on the part of one member of a couple, for whom the defensive nature of the marital fit has become stultifying. Very defensive relationships cannot tolerate the independent development of one partner, since that is seen as a threat to the shared defence. Of course, this is one of the inherent tensions in marriage that I mentioned earlier—autonomy vs. dependency. Where the image of the couple is founded on an idealized fantasy of fusion, the separate development of one partner is felt to threaten the very existence of the marriage. Alternatively, some marriages may allow for the partners to develop outside the relationship, even to the extent of other sexual partners, so long as no pressure is exerted for intimacy *within* the marriage. For them, closeness is as threatening as distance is to the fused couples. Neither of these are successful ways of managing the tension of opposites. However, it is not always possible to tell from the external structure of a marriage what its internal constituents are.

A famous British example is the marriage of Harold Nicholson and Vita Sackville-West, two prominent members of the aristocratic and literary Bloomsbury circle, both of whom had homosexual relationships outside their marriage, lived separately most of the time, and yet stayed together, apparently happily, throughout most of their lives. Both of them were eminently creative, and a biography entitled *Portrait of a Marriage* was later written by their son (Nicholson, 1973). He spoke very positively of this arrangement, and one would have thought he was in a position to know. I include this example as a caution against normative thinking. Individuation by its very nature takes many different forms.

Many couples come to therapy complaining of unequal development, especially when one partner has been in individual therapy, often a more respectable way of making a bid for freedom than having an affair. There are some similarities, since both offer an alternative arena for working at the development of a creative couple: what is enacted concretely and physically in a sexual affair can be worked at symbolically and psychologically within the two-some of therapy. For it is not the unequal development itself that is the problem so much as the failure to contain the resulting tension within the marriage.

Mr and Mrs York requested marital therapy after Mrs York had been in individual therapy for some years. She very much wished to stay in the marriage but felt that unless she could find a way of communicating more openly with her husband, this would be impossible.

Mr York was devastated. He did not want to change individually, feeling that he had reached a workable equilibrium in himself following a breakdown some years earlier. He felt that his wife was intent on disrupting that equilibrium, and he was intent on resisting her. She had suffered a number of serious losses in childhood and was intent on re-working them. He, while initially supportive, had become impatient with the extent and intensity of her quest.

The structure of the relationship appeared to demand that one should be "in" while the other was "out". In the lead-up to his breakdown, Mr York had led an increasingly secretive life outside the home. At that time and following the breakdown Mrs York felt she carried the entire burden of nurturing the relationship between them. In recent years the situation had reversed—Mrs York was leading a "secret" life with her therapist, and Mr York was voicing the need for togetherness.

This split served the function of maintaining distance between them while ensuring that the relationship survived. Now, however, Mrs York was demanding her "secret" life inside the marriage, and this seemed to make demands on Mr York that he was not willing to meet. He, too, had suffered early losses but was very reluctant to re-open the sealed compartment in himself where he had put them. But this part of himself was exactly what Mrs York was seeking access to—the part that could share her own sense of loss with her.

For a long time we as their therapists could not tell whether Mrs York was voicing the need for change on

behalf of both of them or whether hers was a lone voice
that would eventually break the marriage. They used us as
the only place where the conflict could be contained, and it
was only when we interpreted their wish to make us into a
substitute family that the situation shifted. They were
attempting to deny the temporary nature of the
containment we offered, and our interpretation provided a
means of working through their feared losses in the
transference, so that they could eventually relinquish us
and take over the function that we had temporarily
provided. At the point we ended with them, after two years
of marital therapy, Mrs York's individual therapy was still
continuing, but the couple had reached a much better
accommodation. Mr York had, despite himself, worked
through some of his feelings about loss and breakdown
but had also won the right to maintain his equilibrium
relatively undisturbed. Mrs York had won the right to
pursue her individual quest outside the marriage but had
had to recognize that her husband's way was different
from her own. In short, they had reached an
understanding that enabled them to contain the tension of
their differences whilst still acknowledging what they
shared.

Marriage as a container

A marriage that is functioning well offers its participants a form
of containment analogous to the containment that the mother
provides for her infant. In Bion's model, to which I refer at
greater length in "Marriage as a Psychological Container" (chapter five, this volume), the mother receives the infant's unmanageable tensions by means of projective identification. Her
capacity to reflect on what is troubling her baby, which Bion
calls her "reverie", enables her to detoxify these projections and
return them to the infant in a modified and manageable form
(Bion, 1962b). The therapist is called upon to perform much the
same function. Indeed, it is arguable that Bion's model is actually an artificial reconstruction of what takes place in infancy

based on his experience as a psychoanalyst. However, my own
experience as a parent does certainly overlap with my experience as a therapist. Here again containment seems to be about
the capacity to manage the tension of opposites. As a parent
and as a therapist, one provides a bounded space within which
spontaneous processes of growth can take place. Patients, like
children, need protection from the demands and impingements
of the outside world in order to have the freedom to find their
own way at their own pace.

A container is an apt metaphor for this provision. It is symbolized in the sealed vessel of alchemy, the *vas hermeticum*—a
place in which mysterious chemical transformations take
place, which, as Jung has shown, were to be understood properly as spiritual and psychological rather than as concrete
physical events concerned with the transmutation of base matter into gold. "Our gold is not the vulgar gold", runs an old
alchemical motto (Jung, 1944). But the container is more than
the provision of space. It also has an active element, the process of detoxification and modification. It refers not only to the
vessel itself, but to what is going on inside it. When the mother
is required to contain the infant's hate, she must be able to
hold on to the capacity for love; when the infant feels he is
dying, the mother must maintain her belief in the life-giving
milk that flows from her breasts and from her love; when the
infant is in despair, she must hold onto her ability to hope. At
bottom she must believe in her capacity simply to keep going—
to survive, as Winnicott says. But this survival is more than
mere physical survival—it is the survival of the capacity for
thought and reflection, the ability to remain psychically alive in
the face of what can be a very considerable emotional battering.

Containment may also take different forms at different
stages. For the baby, an aggressive response may be shatter-
ing, but for the growing child who is testing out the limits of his
own aggression it may be perfectly appropriate. The parent who
shouts at the child to "stop it at once" is letting him know his
attack has been received and that the parent is confident in the
belief that the conflict will not destroy them.

This last point also makes the connection to the containing
function of marriage. Rows may be unpleasant, but if the couple can maintain their belief in the continuity of their relation-

ship, they are tolerable. There are few things more obviously uncontaining than trying to have a row with a partner who will not respond.

Some couples are so threatened by the prospect of a break in their fragile marital container that they cannot test out its strength at all. In this case the containment provided is of a purely defensive kind. Its purpose is to keep elements sealed off, not so they can unfold in safety within the container, but so that what is outside the container is kept safe from what is within it. The image of this sort of containment is not a chemical retort, but a prison. (As I was writing this, this country was being given a nasty demonstration of the dangers of this sort of containment in the shape of the most brutal, violent, and protracted prison riot the country has ever known.) One couple described the explosive forces that were released by the husband's affair as like being hit in the face by a Jack-in-the-box.

Other couples may be able to get into the dangerous areas but still feel that the marriage is put at risk by them.

Mr and Mrs Norton have suffered for years from periodic outbursts from Mrs Norton, which result in periods of estrangement of up to several weeks. In-between they have a marriage that feels viable, but when the barriers go up, they regularly consider separation. There is a lot of talk from Mrs Norton about how to keep the loving going, while he says he would be happy never to have a row again. He is noticeably uncontaining when his wife has one of these outbursts. Mr Norton becomes quiet and perplexed and never gives her the reassurance that he, too, is capable of violent feelings. The lack of containment tends to make her spiral out of control very quickly: she is capable of moving from a cross word to having her bags packed and ready to go within the space of an hour. In relation to their therapists they are always friendly and reasonable, never showing any signs of frustration or disappointment. This, amongst other signs, has given us the clue to their intense fear of hatred, which is felt to completely wipe out the loving feelings. They long for more of the same, when what they really need is the capacity to sustain both love and hatred. We are providing a therapeutic container that makes possible both the safe expression of hatred—having their row in the session was a big step forward—and the experience that such emotions can be thought about. We are working with them towards their being able to internalize the therapeutic containment into their relationship in the same way that the infant internalizes the mother's containing function.

This is the beginning of the capacity for internal marriage, since what is internalized is a relationship in which there is both a container and a contained. There is, however, a crucial step to be made from the mother-infant relationship to the internal marriage, and this occurs via the relationship that the child has to the parental marriage.

To conclude this discussion of marriage as a container, I would like to indicate what it is not. Many couples who, in terms of their psychic development, have never fully made the transition from the nursing couple to the copulating couple attempt to set up a marriage on the model of parent and child. Of course, there has to be room for this in every marriage—we all need to care and be cared for, and a marriage without the unpredictable spontaneity of the child would be dull indeed. But I am referring to marriages where this is the dominant interaction. Jung referred to this arrangement as the marriage of the container and the contained (Jung, 1925). Although he used the term in a quite different sense to Bion's, it is, I am sure, significant that he chose the same word. He described the way the contained works on the container—like a room that is too small. Unable to find containment themselves, one partner ends up "spying out of the window", while the contained one, feeling the insecurity of their containment, clings on and attempts to push further into the container. A familiar vicious circle: the more one clings, the more the other withdraws.

In "Individuation in Marriage", Lyons and Mattinson (chapter six, this volume), point out that the conscious container is often the unconscious contained and vice versa, especially in those situations where one partner is carrying a double dose. The couple with the black bedroom are a case in point. Several years older than his wife, it was clear that the husband had treated her as a child throughout the marriage. Yet it was she who spied out of the window because of the pressure of having to contain his unconscious dependency as well as her own.

This "spying out of the window" points up the ultimately defensive nature of marriages in which one partner contains the other. At best it is likely to result in the contained eventually getting what they need and flying the nest, having outgrown the relationship. The creative marital container, by contrast, refers not to a function fulfilled by one partner but to a function of the relationship itself—the shared image of a creative internal couple.

Finally, I would like to refer to the development of my own thinking on this subject. I first began thinking about containment in marriage because I felt it provided a bridging concept between defensive and developmental marriages. I was interested in the variety of accommodations that people make, which seemed to be on a continuum between the two—that perhaps for some people a defensive arrangement might prove very successful in enabling them to function well within a limited area. On the other hand I felt that the notion of the developmental marriage was too idealized—I could not see that marriage, while being a therapeutic institution, could have the same therapeutic potential as therapy itself.

However, I have now changed my view. I have realized that development does not mean the putting right of what was felt to be wrong in the past, the re-working of infantile conflicts to the point of resolution. This now seems to me to be an omnipotent expectation. Instead, I have come to see development in terms of the creative tensions of opposites, as I have been discussing in this chapter: something that is going on all the time and is moving forward into the future as well as referring back towards repairing the past. For the individual and for the couple it requires a stable and flexible structure, which is capable of both responding to change and initiating it. Marriage does not have to be the place where I can entirely be myself, but it can be the place where I discover some of the possibilities for becoming myself.

CHAPTER EIGHT

The impenetrable other: ambivalence and the oedipal conflict in work with couples

James Fisher

Oedipal themes

In Freud's view, the pivotal struggle in the human drama centres around what he came to call the Oedipus complex. As Hanna Segal has observed, it contains "the central cluster of conflicting impulses, phantasies, anxieties and defences" and therefore is "the centre of psychoanalytic work" (Segal, 1989). It is hardly surprising that in psychoanalytic psychotherapy with couples there should be an interest in oedipal conflicts.

It is also true that some version of the oedipal drama has become commonplace in contemporary popular culture. Many couples who come for therapy, for example, have a view about how each may have been, in some degree, looking for the parent of the opposite sex in the choice of partners. That does not necessarily represent an awareness of Freud's theories, though it might, but more a kind of popular psychology one might hear in the pub or in the market. It is also not an "insight" that makes any therapeutic difference.

For example, one couple, Lauren and Richard, who came to the Tavistock Institute of Marital Studies for marital therapy had constructed their shared interpretation of their marital conflict around a version of the oedipal story. Lauren, having recently left a professional career at 29 to attend university for the first time, had also left the marital home for student accommodation, because she could no longer tolerate a sexual relationship with her husband. Richard, a successful professional in his mid-30s, had encouraged her to go to university, and he continued to maintain their family home in spite of her desertion of the marital bed.

They saw each other perhaps once a week at most, when they came for therapy. She talked about their relationship like that of a father and daughter, and he, somewhat puzzled, agreed. They were both desperate, unable to part but equally unable to resume their sexual relationship. Though they said they wanted it to be different, they had in fact sustained this apparently unsatisfactory arrangement for 18 months when they came for therapy. They could laugh at themselves, but only with a sense of helplessness.

Peter Gay, in his biography of Freud, highlights the macabre humour that sometimes attaches itself to the oedipal conflict. He cites a caricature of contemporary popular views in the 1920s of psychoanalytic theory by the Hungarian playwright and wit, Ferenc Molnár. Molnár tells us of a plot summary for a proposed play.

> "How this is to be developed," he said, "I don't yet know. But the fundamental idea is quite simple, as in all great tragedies. We have a young man—happily married to his mother. He discovers that she isn't his mother at all. He shoots himself." [Gay, 1988]

Of course, one psychoanalytic view of the therapeutic challenge in working with this couple, Richard and Lauren, is that the work should focus on the so-called "pre-oedipal" issues. The apparently all-too-available oedipal dynamics simply mask these more "primitive" conflicts. In fact, it is possible to work for some time with couples or with individuals psycho-therapeutically without focusing on oedipal issues, perhaps never thinking of the dynamics of the therapy as betraying underlying oedipal conflicts. For example, we might think of this couple as evidencing the considerable difficulty each has in separating from a parental attachment and each as engaged in a consequent struggle for individuation. They may think of it as "oedipal", but in what sense does it suggest a triangular conflict?

Edna O'Shaughnessy makes the invisibility of the Oedipus complex her central theme in a paper in which she suggests that the fact that there appear to be long periods of analysis, or even *whole* analyses, where there is little or no oedipal material could be understood to mean the oedipal issues are unimportant. It may also be that the Oedipus complex is "so important and felt (for whatever reasons) to be so unnegotiable" that "psychic means" are employed "to make and keep it invisible" (O'Shaughnessy, 1989).

My special interest in this chapter is the exploration of some of the primitive dynamics of the oedipal dilemma, which often escape identification as part of that drama, especially in our work with couples. These dynamics bear the scars of a tragically miscarried process, and this is one reason why they are often unrecognized as being shaped by an oedipal conflict. The result in therapy may be a powerful impulse for the drama to be *enacted* rather than to be examined and understood. This "acting out" in the therapy can be, I believe, one of the principal marks of the presence of an unrecognized oedipal drama—an "acting out" by the couple, with consequent pressure on the therapists to participate in the enactment of an unresolved oedipal conflict.

In this chapter I want to provide some brief theoretical and historical background to the evolution of our understanding of the oedipal conflict, suggesting that, beginning with Freud himself, there has been an increasing focus on ambivalence as the central dilemma of the Oedipus complex. In the second half of the chapter, I link this focus on ambivalence with some recent thinking about working with primitive oedipal material that draws on some of Bion's theoretical contributions. I attempt throughout to relate these theoretical explorations with clinical material, to illustrate how this understanding of oedipal conflict can inform therapy with couples who present with this dilemma of the impenetrable other.

In brief, the central theses of this chapter are the following:

1. The capacity to be an individual, to be separate and hence capable of a relationship with another, rests on mastering the anxieties of the triangle. In brief, these are the anxieties, on the one hand, of being excluded from a couple, and, on the other, those of being part of a couple that excludes the third. The mastering of these anxieties results in a sense of psychological space. Conversely, the failure to master these anxieties is experienced as a desperate lack of a sense of psychological or emotional space—space to think, to be different and separate, space in which to enter or leave a relationship.

2. These anxieties and their resolution are intimately linked to those associated with the experience of ambivalence, the feelings of love and hate directed towards the same person.

3. These anxieties are only ever resolved provisionally, *never finally*, and they are commonly, and sometimes even dramatically, revived in the intimacy of a couple relationship. For this reason they are characteristic of many presentations for help by couples having difficulties with their relationships.

Changing views of the Oedipus complex

Freud's exposition of the oedipal conflict traditionally focused on castration anxiety. This is a correlate of his preoccupation with the male genital during what he termed the *phallic* phase of the sexual development of both girls and boys, a phase in which there is "not a primacy of the genitals, but a primacy of the phallus" (Freud, 1923e). It is the prohibition by the father experienced as the threat of castration that leads the little boy to give up his hopes for a sexual relationship with the mother. This, however, is only half of the story—what has come to be

called the "positive" oedipal relationship. There is another side
to the story.

> Closer study usually discloses the more complete Oedipus
> complex, which is twofold, positive and negative, and is due
> to the bisexuality originally present in children: that is to
> say, a boy has not merely an ambivalent attitude towards
> his father and an affectionate object-relation towards his
> mother, but at the same time he also . . . displays an affec-
> tionate *feminine* attitude to his father and a corresponding
> hostility and jealousy towards his mother. [Freud, 1923b,
> italics added]

Should the little boy be successful in his oedipal desires for
mother, he would jeopardize another important affectional attachment, that to his father. Were we to fail to consider the so-
called "negative" Oedipus complex—and the recounting of the
story often does stop here—we would fail to see the basis for the
boy's ambivalent attachment to mother.

Freud is clear about the point, in theory at least, ascribing
the "intricacy of the problem" to two factors: "the triangular
character of the Oedipus situation and the constitutional bi-
sexuality of each individual" (Freud, 1923b).

In fact, Freud seemed to have had some personal resistance
to sustaining this aspect of the oedipal conflict in his discussions. Peter Gay, for example, points out that the only emotional tie Freud "sentimentalized" was that of the mother's love
for her son (Gay, 1988). While every lasting intimate relationship, whether in marriage, friendship, or the family, conceals a
sediment of hostile feelings, according to Freud, there is perhaps "one single exception," the "relation of mother to son"
(Freud, 1921c). He put it most enthusiastically in the *New Introductory Lectures*: "This is altogether the most perfect, the
most free from ambivalence of all human relationships" (Freud,
1933a).

Meltzer notes that for Freud the Rat Man case represented a
"significant historical landmark" in that here for the first time
he used the concept of ambivalence and recognized it as the
possible basis for neurosis (Meltzer, 1978). In fact, ambivalence
had also figured in the case of Little Hans (Freud, 1909b).
Nevertheless, in his later work in the 1920s Freud placed

greater emphasis on ambivalence—for example, in his discussion of little Hans' oedipal dilemma in *Inhibitions, Symptoms and Anxiety* (1926d [1925]):

> He was at the time in the jealous and hostile Oedipus attitude towards his father, whom nevertheless—except in so far as his mother was the cause of estrangement—he dearly loved. Here, then, we have a conflict due to ambivalence: a well-grounded love and a no less justified hatred directed towards one and the same person.

Freud then goes on to a discussion of various defensive manoeuvres for dealing with ambivalence, such as repression, reaction-formation, displacement, and the relationship of these defences to symptom formation. Though he notes the centrality of ambivalence in the oedipal dilemma and makes clear how this calls for some way of coping, presumably because the ambivalence is felt to be intolerable, he nevertheless returns to fear as the central motive for the resolution of this conflict—the fear of castration. One might almost see that as a *paranoid* retreat from the dilemma of ambivalence and itself perhaps therefore more a *defence against* it.

While it is important to recognize the powerful effect of the castration threat in the oedipal drama, it is also important to note that at best it would only provide a plausible motive for the resolution of the boy's "positive" oedipal complex. If we take into account the "negative" oedipal dilemma, we are forced to widen our consideration of the core anxieties. Freud, too, faced this problem, as can be seen when we come to consider the situation of the little girl. As he put it: "Whereas in boys the Oedipus complex is destroyed by the castration complex, in little girls it is made possible and led up to by the castration complex" (Freud, 1925j). In other words, castration anxiety fails to account adequately for the giving up of oedipal wishes in the little girl and, I suggest, in the little boy in his "negative" oedipal dilemma.

Freud's solution in reference to the little girl was to develop a convoluted, changing account of her Oedipus complex. The core anxiety for her was described as the fear of the loss of love, which must include both the loss of the loved object and the loss of the love of the object.

Since, however, most of his attempts to describe the course of the oedipal drama for the girl did not put the emphasis on the dilemma of ambivalence, Freud was left in the end with the conclusion that "in girls the motive for the demolition of the Oedipus complex is lacking" (Freud, 1925j). This led him inevitably, though he says *hesitantly*, to the conclusion that "for women the level of what is ethically normal is different from what it is in men" (Freud, 1925j).

I cannot resist a brief aside here about a matter that deserves a chapter of its own. Freud has a seriously attenuated basis for a theory of moral experience, his theory of what he calls the "superego". Founding morality on the castration threat, Freud leaves women no basis for moral experience and men with a morality based on fear of punishment. It is only by following Freud's hints concerning the centrality of ambivalence in the oedipal drama that we see how there could be an empirical grounding for a moral theory based on concern for the other.

What is perhaps most striking for our purposes here is Freud's gradual appreciation in his later works of the centrality of ambivalence as a major—indeed, universal—focus of conflict and consequent anxiety. His attention during this period focused to a large extent on the duality of the death and life instincts, a theoretical and somewhat metaphysical way, I suggest, of exploring the experience of ambivalence.

Even as late as 1931, however, Freud was expressing what we might call his own ambivalence about *ambivalence*. On the one hand he was increasingly recognizing its core importance. On the other hand, in 1931 he argued that ambivalence was an *archaic trait*, associated with "primitive races" and the "first phases of erotic life". *Normal* adults, as the result of later developments, he says, succeed in separating love and hatred *and do not find themselves obliged to hate their love-objects and to love their enemy as well as to hate him* (Freud, 1931b; italics added).

This 1931 paper is especially interesting because in it Freud comes to an increasing emphasis on the "activity" as well as the "passivity" in the little girl in the evolution of her Oedipus complex. That is, we must continuously keep in mind the so-called "negative" as well as the "positive" oedipal conflict. In

the end he agrees with Lampl-de-Groot (1927) when he concludes that, "the whole development is summed up in the for-
mula that the girl goes through a phase of the 'negative'
Oedipus complex before she can enter the positive one" (Freud,
1931b). At this stage of his career Freud was no longer engaged
in intensive clinical work and thus had no real opportunity to
continue this exploration to its logical end.

In my view Freud comes closest to the emotional heart of
the matter in his last publication in 1940, when he again discusses the nature of the castration anxiety. He had already
described, in his paper on "The Dissolution of the Oedipus
Complex", how the child must in the end turn away from the
hopeless longing because of the experience of painful disappointments. It is a case not just of the threat of castration but,
more importantly, of its *internal impossibility*" (Freud, 1924d).

In his *An Outline of Psychoanalysis* (1940a [1938]), his last
publication, Freud makes clearer than he had ever done before
the "painful impossibility" at the core of the experience for the
boy *and* for the mother—a painful impossibility that is, perhaps, to give Freud the benefit of a metaphorical interpretation,
inevitably a kind of cruel "castration":

> When a boy (from the age of two or three) has entered the
> phallic phase of his libidinal development, is feeling pleas-
> urable sensations in his sexual organ and has learnt to
> procure these at will by manual stimulation, he becomes
> his mother's lover. He wishes to possess her physically in
> such ways as he has divined from his observations and
> intuitions about sexual life, and he tries to seduce her by
> showing her the male organ which he is proud to own. . . .
>
> The boy's mother has understood quite well that his sexual
> excitation relates to herself. Sooner or later she reflects that
> it is not right to allow it to continue. She thinks she is doing
> the correct thing in forbidding him to handle his genital
> organ.

Here we see clearly that it is not some cultural or social norm
operating in the castration threat but, rather, a profound emotional dilemma, a dilemma in the first instance for the mother,
but by extension, through her relationship with her partner, a
dilemma for the parental couple. It is not a matter of some

"enlightened" or "unenlightened" attitude towards infantile sexuality. It is the painfully tragic erotic attachment that reaches across a chasm, a chasm created by the inexorable difference between the generations, by the reality of the difference between the experience of being the parent and the experience of being the child. In this sense questions about the universality of the oedipal conflict are misconstrued. Nothing could be more universal than the difference between the generations (see Simon, 1991).

Mother's own sexual feelings are aroused in what she must finally acknowledge as an impossible link. Of course it is not literally impossible, as Oedipus and Jocasta knew. But to cross that line is to *pervert*, not to erase, the reality of the difference between the generations. The core of the oedipal and, we should hasten to add, of the Jocastan tragedy is that feelings do cross that divide. And they lead to a dilemma from which there is no painless escape, except by self-crippling illusions or an attack on the psychic apparatus itself and its capabilities (Britton, 1989).

The capacity for relationship is grounded in the capacity for tolerating this *impossible* dilemma of the oedipal triangle, as I hope to show in the next section. Ironically, it is the triadic relationship that provides the basis for a dyadic relationship, not the other way around. This is an even stronger version of Blos's interesting challenge to the traditional notion that the resolution of dyadic relationships is necessary to the establishment of triadic ones (Blos, 1985).

Discussions of Melanie Klein's revisions of Freud's account of the Oedipus complex often focus on her earlier dating of the appearance of this triangular conflict. But, I suggest, the more important aspect of her account is the emphasis on the centrality of ambivalence as the core conflict. The resolution of the conflict, it follows, lies with the ability to tolerate and not to avoid or evade that painful ambivalence. In short-hand, it is the experience of what Klein came to call the "depressive position"—that is, the capacity for acknowledging the hated and the loved object as one and the same.

Britton spells this out in his argument that working through the Oedipus complex entails working through the depressive position.

The oedipal rivalry both in the positive (heterosexual) form and in the negative (homosexual) form provides a means of working through the depressive position. In each version one parent is the object of desire, and the other is the hated rival. This configuration is retained, but the feeling changes in relation to each parent. Thus good becomes bad and vice-versa as positive changes to negative. My contention is that the evasive use of this switch is halted by the full recognition of the parents' sexual relationship, their different anatomy, and the child's own nature. This involves the realisation that the same parent who is the object of oedipal desire in one version is the hated rival in the other. [Britton, 1989]

In this view of the Oedipus complex, what moves to the fore is the centrality of the parental relationship, the knowledge and the phantasies about the parental couple. As Britton points out, what is required is a recognition that the parents' relationship is genital and procreative and the parent–child relationship is not. "This recognition produces a sense of loss and envy, which if not tolerated, may become a sense of grievance or self-denigration" (Britton, 1989). The question is, how does one come to tolerate the intolerable?

The impenetrable other

One of the couples that led me to thinking about the dynamics of *the impenetrable other*—I shall call them Carol and Martin—referred themselves to the Tavistock Institute of Marital Studies in a state of crisis.

Martin was desperate because Carol had, without his knowledge, arranged to take their two young children to her home country without telling him. He had only found out about it at the last moment and had hidden their passports, so they could not go. He was in a panic over what seemed to him collusion between Carol and her mother to exclude him from any part in what would happen to his two children, to whom he was devoted. In his application for marital therapy he had included a copy of a four-page closely hand-written letter, which, he said, he had sent to his mother-in-law.

The letter was typical of Martin's desperate way of trying to get through to someone he felt could not or would not understand him.

The letter did not make you want to read it, and in fact in the intake process virtually no one who looked through the application forms read the letter, although it contained vital information. Because it went on and on and on, it failed to engage the reader. Martin was well aware of this difficulty of his. He described himself as trying to be reasonable and restrained in communicating with Carol. However, when she did not respond, which he felt was all of the time now, he found himself going on and on with her in a way that was futile and even counterproductive. He knew it was useless, but he could not help himself. And he frequently enacted this in the sessions, not only with Carol, but also with my co-therapist and myself, filling the session with his orations but leaving us feeling that we understood nothing.

When we tried to explore this with Martin, he became prickly and even openly paranoid. He would then withdraw into a sulk. It was as difficult for us to get through to him as it was for him to get through to us. Words often felt like missiles that were to be fended off rather than some means of communication and understanding.

Carol's experience in the marriage was as desperate. Nothing she did was right. Martin was controlling down to the smallest detail of cleaning the house or dealing with the children. She felt he never listened to her, and she felt bombarded and helpless. Unable to tolerate his harangues, she began to shut herself off. She simply did not respond. The result, not surprisingly, was an explosion.

One of the main complaints about their relationship from both Carol and Martin was that they did not have enough space. They described this graphically in terms of their physical living space, which mirrored their emotional state. They lived in a small house—one bedroom and bath upstairs, a sitting room and tiny kitchen downstairs. She lived upstairs, he downstairs. In fact, because of his music, there was no comfortable furniture in the "sitting room", and it had become more of a chaotic "studio". There was no sense of a shared space at all. Even in the only room where the whole family gathered occasionally when awake, the kitchen, Martin sat literally in the doorway into the other room.

The sessions reproduced this uncannily. There was no space to think and understand, no space for a relationship between them or between them and me and my co-therapist. Either Martin was holding forth and Carol remote, or there was an explosion. When there was an explosion, it reverberated up and down the corridor, making our couple for a time infamous in the TIMS.

OR there was something that *seemed* different but in fact illustrated the fragility of any attempt to share. At the first session following a long summer break, there was considerable tentativeness all around, though they mentioned nothing about the explosion during a threesome just before the break. Carol talked for almost the whole of the session, engaged primarily in a dialogue with me. Towards the end of the session we tried to explore a little the meaning of Martin's silence. He said he felt it was important for Carol to talk and was afraid that, if he joined in, he would spoil it.

It was only after the session, when my co-therapist talked about how excluded she had felt, that we could begin to understand something of the pervasive anxiety. She knew she felt excluded but felt that if she commented on that or tried to make a link with Martin's experience, she would spoil what was going on.

This did not mean that there existed a real couple—real in the sense that it was robust enough to tolerate feelings of exclusion *or* conversely the feelings associated with being part of a couple that excluded others. It was as if we were all holding our breath. For the first time, Carol was talking about her feeling that somehow *she* was the one who spoiled therapy any time she became honestly involved. There was a palpable fear that if we could engage with those feelings, somehow it would all explode again.

One of the most important developments in recent psycho-analytic theory has been a theory that offers a way of thinking about the process through which the infant can learn to toler-ate the overwhelming fears and anxieties to which it is subject. It was Bion who introduced the notion of the "container/con-tained" relationship to describe an interaction between the in-fant and mother in which the mother is able, unconsciously, to experience traumatic feelings that the infant finds unbear-able. In interaction with a mother able to tolerate these feel-ings in herself, the infant, too, comes to experience them as bearable.

In his description of this process, Bion makes use of the Kleinian notion of projective identification—in the first instance a powerful projective defence *against* anxiety, but in Bion's view also an essential developmental relationship (Bion, 1962a, 1967, 1970). In their recent elaborations of the Oedipus com-plex, Britton, Feldman, and O'Shaughnessy (Steiner, 1989) all make use of Bion's notion of "container/contained", emphasiz-ing it as an important developmental factor not only in the relationship to the mother, but also in the relationship to the parental couple. This aspect of the dynamic of "containment" in Bion's sense is of critical importance for work with couples.

One way to get some idea of the meaning of containment is to turn for a moment to Winnicott's description of what he calls the "good-enough mother" and his related notion of the "false self". In fact, the couple I have described at some length, Martin and Carol, illustrate what we might think of as the two sides of the interactional experience that leads to the false self organization. Winnicott describes this in the first instance in terms of his notion of the "good-enough mother"—the mother sufficiently able to respond to the spontaneous gestures of the infant. The mother's "relatively successful adaptation to the infant's gestures and needs" leads to the infant's experience of its omnipotence as somehow magically linked to what becomes understood eventually as external reality. The infant that has an experience of a mother unable sufficiently to do this may then cope through compliance. As Winnicott puts it, the "not-good-enough mother" "substitutes her own gesture which is to be given sense by compliance of the infant" (Winnicott, 1960b).

We need a complementary term for the "false self"—a term that refers to the infant as mother's object, the compliant object. A list of possible synonyms is itself quite suggestive: obedient, amenable, submissive, passive, yielding, acquiescent, docile, meek. What I am suggesting is that the pressure of the gesture of the "not-good-enough mother" can be experienced as a demand to fit in and thus sustain what we might call the "false self couple". It often has what seems to be a quite benign form, such as mother's *telling* the infant not to cry, that everything will be all right.

When the false self personality, however, enacts its version of a relationship to the "compliant object" it becomes tyrannical, thus revealing an important hidden dimension of the subjective experience of the false self.

Martin's tyrannical demands of Carol demonstrate in an extreme form the desperation to sustain this "false self couple" in the face of something felt to be intolerable. I suggest that Martin's demands were a manifestation of a false self organization for several reasons. One is the empirical fact that he also described himself, both in his work relationships and in his childhood, as always having to fit in. He had a strong sense that to risk being himself in a spontaneous way is a risk he had never been able take. But there is also a conceptual reason to link what we might think of as the active and passive aspects of compliance, the fitting in or the demand that someone else fit in.

If we ask why it is that mother cannot recognize and respond to the infant's spontaneous gesture, it is worth reflecting on Freud's comments concerning the mother's, perhaps unconscious, recognition of the meaning of the little boy's touching his penis. It cannot be tolerated because of the internal conflicts it raises. And it is not, of course, just the erotic gestures that are difficult to tolerate. As difficult are the furious, raging, and hurtful gestures coming from the infant. The mother who cannot feel contained in the anxiety of her own conflicting feelings will find the infant's anxiety of its conflicting feelings intolerable.

When thinking about Winnicott's notion of the "false self", it is worth going back to his earlier paper, "Hate in the Countertransference" (1947):

> The mother, however, hates her infant from the word go. I believe Freud thought it possible that a mother may in certain circumstances have only love for her boy baby; but we may doubt this. . . .

Winnicott then proceeds to list 18 reasons why a mother hates her baby, "even a boy", and he concludes:

> A mother has to be able to tolerate hating her baby without doing anything about it. . . .

> It seems to me doubtful whether a human child as he develops is capable of tolerating the full extent of his own hate in a sentimental environment. He needs hate to hate.

One way of understanding what happens with the "not-good-enough mother", the mother who cannot tolerate her own conflicting feelings, is that mother's own defensive false self organization takes an active form in gestures towards the infant aimed (no doubt unconsciously) at seducing the infant into a compliance with this false self.

It is interesting that one of the recurrent themes of Martin's badgering of Carol concerned her control of the children. He could hold forth for a whole session on the psychological considerations of how often to tell children to do something before convincing them that you really mean it.

Similarly, there was an almost continuous pressure on my co-therapist and myself to take control, either to stop Martin's dominating a session or to stop their sometimes "unstoppable" rows, or in the face of Carol's impenetrable facade to try to break through to her by pursuing her with questions. It was a seductive pressure to join in an enactment of the *false self couple* in a caricature of therapy.

The essential triangle

It is helpful, I think, to put Winnicott's notion of the false self organization in the context of the oedipal conflict. Winnicott himself notes the essential function of the *other* in the creation of the special relation of the mother to infant which he calls "devotion".

In order to create the mother–infant couple there must be another relationship with mother that is both sustaining and containing and yet capable of being the *other* excluded from this new special couple. In some cultures and social environments this is the husband, in others the mother or mother and sisters. In some cases there has to be a "splitting" by the mother into the responsible *caretaker* on the one hand and on the other the mother lost in devoted reverie with her new-born. The *other* is there from the beginning, as is the potential trauma for the infant in trying to manage the anxieties when the good breast/provider/partner is otherwise occupied.

In a fascinating reading of Shakespeare's *Troilus and Cressida*, Janet Adelman (1985) offers a view of Cressida's "betrayal" as in fact her status as a separate person, something that Troilus finds intolerable. Here we have a clear view of the early triangular crisis.

> At issue here is, I suspect, a primitive fantasy in which separation *is* infidelity: for the infant, the mother's separateness constitutes the first betrayal; insofar as she is not merely his, she is promiscuously other. I suspect that this sense of otherness itself as promiscuous betrayal antedates the more specific oedipal jealousies and is retrospectively sexualized by them. The whole process is condensed in the play's demonstration, in the character of Cressida, that separation, opaque otherness, and sexual betrayal are one.

On the other hand, Klein suggests that it is also the experience of the *good* feeding breast that allows the infant to turn to other (potentially good) objects, mirroring, I think, a phantasy of the good other to whom mother turns (Klein, 1945).

It is important to note that after Klein's formulation of the depressive position, her views of the Oedipus complex altered.

Segal notes that she increasingly saw the two as linked. In the depressive position there is a diminution of paranoid anxieties. By degrees love and concern take the upper hand over the hatred. "Gradually Klein came to the conclusion that the beginnings of the Oedipus complex are not associated with the phase of maximum sadism—an idea she came to discard—but, on the contrary, it is linked with diminishing sadism." Awareness of ambivalence towards both parents and towards their relationship leads to some defensive reaction, for example, regression to splitting and paranoid anxieties as a defence against guilt. "It also brings reparative impulses aimed not only at the restoration of the breast and mother, but also, and increasingly, at restoring a good parental couple and a good family as a whole" (Segal, 1989).

It is this relationship that the infant is desperate to recreate somehow when it feels that its destructive feelings and phantasies have destroyed it in anger and rage. We might even think of Winnicott's "transitional objects" as the infant's experimenting with creating a new couple relationship for itself, something with which it can be preoccupied. The transitional nature of the object has then, perhaps, something to do with the phantasy that this new couple would damage or destroy the other and the defence against this anxiety, hence it can *be* mother or it can *be* the infant's newly created or discovered other, as needed.

It follows that the separation from the primary other, the creation of the space to be an individual, is a process that involves some recognition of the primary couple. Britton's exposition of the function of the triangular relationship as providing the basis for the experience of space is helpful in this regard. He argues that the recognition of the parental relationship creates a boundary for the internal world making possible what he calls a "triangular space". This provides a grounding for the "separation/individuation" process in the oedipal relationship.

> It includes, therefore, the possibility of being a participant in a relationship and observed by a third person as well as being an observer of a relationship between two people. . . . The capacity to envisage a benign parental relationship influences the development of a space outside the self capable of being observed and thought about, which provides

the basis for a belief in a secure and stable world. [Britton, 1989]

Britton goes on to make clear that the experience of ambivalence and the developing capacity for tolerating the anxieties associated with ambivalence are central to this process.

Initially this parental link is conceived in primitive part-object terms and in the modes of [the infant's] hatred expressed in oral, anal and genital terms. If the link between the parents perceived in love and hate can be tolerated in the child's mind, it provides him with a prototype for an object relationship of a third kind in which he is a witness and not a participant. A third position then comes into existence from which object relationships can be observed. Given this, we can also envisage *being* observed. This provides us with a capacity for seeing ourselves in interaction with others and for entertaining another point of view whilst retaining our own, for reflecting on ourselves whilst being ourselves. [Britton, 1989]

We might also say that it is not only that tolerating such a link between the parents provides a "prototype" for a third kind of object relationship but that it is such a link being re-created repeatedly in unconscious phantasy that is the unconscious basis of all creative couplings.

Britton notes that anyone who has worked with a psychotic patient or has been involved in a psychotic transference will appreciate what it means to lack what he is calling that "third position". I want to add that if one has worked with some couples in psychoanalytic therapy, couples that exemplify the dynamic of the *impenetrable other*, that experience will be all too familiar.

Certainly with Martin and Carol there was little possibility for any creative understanding of difference. If either gave an account of anything, the other could not hear out without interrupting to insist that it was not true. It had to be her account or his account, and at times it reached such a pitch that no one could hear anything.

In Bion's exposition of the dynamic of the mother–infant interaction, it is only when the mother is capable of containing the infant's projection of its panic and anxiety that it can begin to learn to tolerate these feelings. When this happens, in Segal's words, "the infant can reintroject his projections, modified by understanding, and he also introjects the breast as a container capable of containing and dealing with anxiety" (Segal, 1989). The failure of containment is in some sense the failure of the integration of the "good" and the "bad".

To the extent that there is failure of this maternal containment, the infant's plight becomes increasingly extreme. Britton argues that in Bion's view, "the inability of the mother to take in her child's projections is experienced *by the child* as a destructive attack *by her* on his link and communication *with her* as his good object" (Britton, 1989, italics added). In other words, both infant and mother are faced, right at the beginning, with what we might describe as the dilemma of the depressive position. The infant that experiences an impermeable mother not able to receive the infant's desperate projections nor able to tolerate its (or her) anxieties has an almost impossible predicament. The good mother (or breast) has become the attacking, destructive mother (breast).

> The idea of a good maternal object can only be regained by splitting off her impermeability so that now a hostile force is felt to exist, which attacks his good link with his mother. Mother's goodness is now precarious and depends on him restricting his knowledge of her. Enlargement of knowledge as a consequence of development and his curiosity are felt to menace this crucial relationship. [Britton, 1989]

Curiosity, which has led inevitably to an awareness of the oedipal relationship—to an awareness of an "other" in mother's field of attention—will then also lead to the possibility that the idea of the "hostile force" may then become identified with the oedipal father. The parental relationship in the infant's phantasy then becomes the arena, and the image of the primal scene becomes the occasion for a disaster.

Bion refers to the disposition to attack the link between two objects, the prototype of which is the link between the mouth and the breast, which arouses the infant's hatred and envy. He suggests that even when the infant is a participant in a creative act, sharing an enviable emotional experience, it is also identified with the excluded party, with the consequent pain, envy, and jealousy. The response of the infant to the experience, or phantasy of the creative link—first between mouth and breast, later between the sexual parents—is attacked and transformed in phantasy into a hostile and destructive sexuality, rendering the couple sterile.

In this chapter, however, I am focusing on Feldman's hypothesis about a similar clinical picture, which, he suggests, has a different underlying dynamic. It has much in common with Britton's exposition of a distorted oedipal development in which there has been a failure of maternal containment.

> The other process I have referred to also results in the patient's experience of the oedipal couple as being engaged in some bizarre and often violent interaction, but it seems to have a different origin and is based on a different mechanism. In this case the infant is not confronted with a creative couple, arousing his envy, but a parental figure or a couple that he finds impenetrable, unable properly to receive or respond to his projections. This may give rise to violent attempts to get through . . . or to a sense of a hopeless and bizarre situation that cannot be faced. . . .
> [Feldman, 1989]

It is not just the impenetrable mother that Feldman is calling attention to. It is also the impenetrable couple. A dream of an individual patient I saw illustrates how this may present in psychoanalytic work.

> This patient presented a particular dilemma in that over a long period of time she had made numerous unsuccessful attempts to get herself into treatment. In spite of her obvious determination to get engaged in therapy, she seemed to be enacting what felt like a desperate "attack" on the therapeutic process. With me this took one of its more dramatic forms in walkouts: seven in the first three years. The therapy felt almost continuously under threat as she tried to purge herself of pain and despair by walking out of the consulting room and in the process

convinced both herself and me that the therapy was at an end.

Over the course of the therapy we came to understand the walkout not merely as an escape from something felt to be intolerable. It was also an "explosion" resulting from her attempt to bring the therapy couple together, as the following dream suggests, and my paralysed silence was a momentary enactment of the desolation created by that explosion.

There was a river, and on either side of the river were two towns. She was on one side with her father, and her mother was on the other side. On the one side were plastic tubes or something like that sticking up. They seemed to her very male, sexual symbols. She tried to cross a bridge to bring the two sides together, to connect them. But then there was an explosion, and everything was destroyed. But it did not matter, because they were all empty houses, desolate, with no sign of human habitation or anything alive anyway.

The parental relationship, in the dream and in my patient's experience of it, was a catastrophe. What I wish to emphasize, however, is her role in it in phantasy, her desperation to bring the two together. Her relationship with an impenetrable mother, depressed, withdrawn (and eventually suffering a cruel degenerative illness), found an echo in her relationship with a sometimes impenetrable therapist. But she did not give up. She was also enacting a phantasy of having some means by which she could magically repair the damage of her attacks in phantasy, trying to bring alive the caring, responsive mother and thus avoiding her sense of unbearable guilt. The second part of the dream illustrates how these were connected by her.

Then she was with other adolescent girls, and they were all being given something. She looked in her envelope and either there was nothing, or at least she could not understand what it was. All the other girls seemed to be pleased with what they had in their envelopes but she had either not been given anything or what it was she could not figure out, could not use.

In this patient's dreams and phantasies the penis either appeared as persecuting and damaging or as "plastic", artificial, and useless. Still there was something in her phantasies that she might have had with which she could have brought the parental couple together in a lively, creative way. As Klein points out:

> Reparative phantasies represent, often in minute detail, the obverse of sadistic phantasies, and to the feeling of sadistic omnipotence corresponds the feeling of reparative omnipotence. . . . Both boy and girl, though in different ways, feel that the penis which damaged and destroyed the mother in their sadistic phantasies becomes the means of restoring and curing her in phantasies of reparation. [Klein, 1945]

My patient experienced both what Feldman describes as "violent attempts to get through" to the impenetrable mother and the impenetrable therapist, as well as, "a sense of a hopeless and bizarre situation" in therapy. But she persisted.

In this she is, I suggest, a model for some types of couples we see in therapy. They present a "bizarre and hopeless" situation in their marriage and demonstrate, both in their relationship and often dramatically in therapy, "violent attempts to get through" to the other and to the therapists. As therapists, we sometimes feel overwhelmed with a sense of despair, especially after a particularly fraught session in which neither seems able to understand what the other says or feels but both persist, almost violently, trying to get through to the other.

This dynamic of the "impenetrable other" takes a variety of guises, though I think it is quite unmistakable.

> Rachel and Michael were, for example, more "civilized" and would courteously let each other have a turn. But the difference in their perceptions of even apparently trivial events was no less profound. Both were highly successful professionals, intelligent and thoughtful, and yet at times it was difficult to believe that for them any experience was a shared experience, or that they could feel sufficient emotional distance to be able to reflect on their different

perceptions in a way that could lead to creative understanding. At times listening to them would make my co-therapist and me think that we must be crazy.

One image that Rachel and Michael provided illustrates the oral dimension of this dilemma. They went to the theatre frequently, they had the best tickets for everything, but they could seldom manage either to arrive together, or to share intervals, or even sometimes to leave together. Despite their best efforts it was difficult to have a shared experience of almost anything they valued. One evening they arrived at the last moment, separately, and found they only had enough money between them to share one cup of coffee and one sandwich. The poverty of what they could share was painful. Sessions were sometimes litanies of their feeling excluded. After one session dominated by the theme of their (shared?) love of making music, my co-therapist suggested that it sounded like a *duet for one*.

This dynamic had a profound effect on the therapist couple as well. For a number of months at the beginning of therapy I found myself irritated and angry with my co-therapist. Michael loved to "hold forth", intellectualizing about himself, their relationship, and about therapy. My co-therapist, so it seemed clearly to me, responded by long interpretations in which she seemed to me to be pursuing them relentlessly, repeating points at length as if trying to force them to understand something.

I sometimes felt excluded, angry that if only we would do it my way, it would be better. I could understand this (intellectually) as some countertransference phenomenon, but it was not until my co-therapist had to miss a session that I really began to understand it. On my own with them, I found myself pursuing this couple relentlessly with long interpretations, as if I had to make them understand but could not. It truly was a duet for one.

The *duet for one* is, I have been suggesting, the *false couple* made up of the *tyrannical self* and the *compliant object*, or, conversely, the *compliant self* and the *tyrannical object*, unable together to create the triangular space necessary for genuine mutual relating.

It should be noted that there is a positive side to this experience of being *one* rather than *two* in a relationship. We could call it the illusion of the *fused couple*. We experienced this with Daniel and Susan, a couple whose intolerance of being together *and* of being apart was even more profound than that of Martin and Carol.

It was Daniel's and Susan's second marriage, and between them they brought seven children to the new relationship. At the time of coming to therapy, they were living separately. The two of them together had moments they described as "idyllic", but the hostility and hatred towards each others' children was as painful to listen to as it was for them to bear. The sessions were explosive, and my co-therapist and I often despaired of getting through a session, let alone through therapy with them.

Immediately after one particularly fraught session, we were just collecting ourselves when several colleagues burst into the room (unheard of in the ethos of the TIMS). What had we done to this couple? They were going down the corridor arm-in-arm in this most idyllic loving state. What was our "magic"? Some time later Daniel and Susan told us that this idyllic state happened frequently. They felt this blissful "togetherness" immediately after a session. The phantasy of the "blissful union" is a complementary aspect of the dynamics of the impenetrable other. Needless to say, this manic union did not last very long. Each wanted to be loved—"warts and all", to use Daniel's phrase—something much more profound than this idyllic illusion. These fleeting idyllic states, exciting though they were, did not mean they could share a life together. They only meant they could not part.

These clinical examples point towards some of the ways in which the *impenetrable other* couples exert a powerful pressure on the therapists to join in enacting rather than understanding in the therapy session. They present considerable technical difficulties as we struggle to try to find the space to reflect on what is happening in the session. To explore this in any detail would take us beyond the limits of this chapter. Nevertheless, I want to make one observation in conclusion.

Meltzer comments on the difficulty in working with individuals who present with the false self or "pseudo-mature" organization. "So skilled is the counterfeiting of maturity in thought, attitude, communication, and action that *only the dreams* make possible this teasing apart of infantile "pseudo-mature" items from the adult pattern of life" (Meltzer, 1966, italics added).

It is sometimes thought that psychoanalytic work with couples cannot "tease apart" these deeply unconscious configurations—dreams, for example, not being a major feature of the presented material. That may be, but it is not because the unconscious hides its traces so well. In fact, it was Meltzer, and others following him, who called our attention to the presence of the unconscious in the session with the notion of "acting in" (Meltzer, 1967). I would suggest that the regressive pull of the couple relationship frequently produces sessions that resemble nothing so much as enacted dreams—dreams, which we as therapists are under persistent pressure to join in acting out that central crisis in human experience, the oedipal drama, dreams of yet another *duet for one* or an encounter with yet another impenetrable other.

CHAPTER NINE

Betrayal of troth

Janet Mattinson

During my working life as a marital psychotherapist, I believe I was able, like most natural or well-trained therapists, to accept and give the necessary space to my patients' feelings of distress, fear, disbelief, anger, or frustration when their partner had been unfaithful to them or their trust had been abused or misused in some way. I was within a few years of my retirement from marital psychotherapy when I became consciously aware of the importance of the archetypal theme of betrayal and its persistent influence on the behaviour of married couples seeking help with their troubled marriage. I write this sentence with shame. I would, no doubt, have been more aware than I had been if I had worked with couples in a Divorce Court Welfare or Conciliation Service, after the final separation had taken place. On the whole I was working with couples who wanted to repair and make their marriage work, albeit often very ambivalently so. I now believe that we do our married or separated patients a disservice if we do not consciously relate to and refer to their feeling of having been betrayed by their partner.

167

In taking our cue from their particular expression of feeling, we need to link their unique experience of betrayal with our own wider understanding of its salience in the experience of mankind. There is little written directly about this theme in the technical psychological texts, but because of its constant recurrence in the large events of the history of the world and in the day-to-day behaviour of all men and women, it has been well recorded in myth, fable, and legend, by historians and in so many classical and modern works of fiction.

Let us just remind ourselves of some old and modern tales. First, a fable:

> An Ass and a Fox went into partnership and sallied out to forage for food together. They hadn't gone far before they saw a Lion coming their way, at which they were both dreadfully frightened. But the Fox thought he saw a way of saving his own skin and went boldly up to the Lion and whispered in his ear, "I'll arrange that you shall get hold of the Ass without the trouble of stalking him, if you'll promise to let me go free". The Lion agreed to this, and the Fox then rejoined his companion and contrived before long to lead him by a hidden pit, which some hunter had dug as a trap for wild animals, and into which he fell. When the Lion saw that the Ass was safely caught and couldn't get away, it was to the Fox that he first turned his attention, and he soon finished him off, and then at his leisure proceeded to feast upon the Ass. [Aesop]

There are many stories of betrayal in the Old Testament: to name but a few, there are those of Samson and Delilah; Cain and Abel; Jacob and Esau; Joseph sold by his brothers and his father deceived; Pharaoh's broken promise; and Tamar's vengeance of Judah. In the New Testament, Judas' betrayal of Jesus was done with a kiss and for thirty pieces of silver. Despite Peter's protestations that never would he betray the Lord, Jesus replied, "This night before the cock crow, thou shalt deny me thrice".

If we turn back to the history books, we can recall Isabella's betrayal of Edward II. Shakespeare reconstructed the story of Anthony and Cleopatra, and of Julius Caesar and Brutus. Betrayal is the hallmark of all his tragedies.

Hamlet, it will be remembered, felt totally betrayed by his mother's apparent forgetfulness of his father by her hasty marriage to Claudius, long before his father's ghost told him of foul murder. And let us remind ourselves of the hell devoted to traitors in Dante's *Divine Comedy*.

More recent literature is as studded with the theme as is the classical. In all of E. M. Forster's novels it is a *leitmotif*. At the beginning of *A Passage to India* (1924), Mrs Moore is almost too good to be true. To both Adela and Dr Aziz, she is a person to be trusted and to be depended upon when they need her most. Then she abandons them and refuses her help. Forster suggests that she does this only when she herself has experienced utter abandonment in the Marabar caves. The false self of the perfect mother, her previously cherished image of herself, broke down. She was left, in Forster's words, with "the underlying worm itself, incapable of generosity". She knew about the echo in the cave, but she said to Adela, "If you don't know, you don't know. I can't tell you."

In modern fiction the theme continues to occur. In Penelope Lively's *The Road to Lichfield* (1977), Mr Stanaway turns and looks at his wife. "I am sorry", he says, "that I seem to have kept something of myself back from you. That is, perhaps, the shabbiest betrayal of all."

In Deborah Moggach's *Porky* (1983), Heather says, "In the end it is consistency you want in people, not perfection. Betrayal is to find them do what you would not have expected. Just that." Also writing about searing childhood memories, betrayal, and cruelty in *Cat's Eye* (1989), the Canadian author Margaret Attwood, speaking through the voice of Elaine when describing one facet of her relationship with her brother, tells how, "We fight in whispers . . . because if we're caught we will both be punished. For this reason we don't tell on each other. We know from experience that the satisfactions of betrayal are scarcely worth it." And she never tells of the treachery of her so-called friend, Cordelia, who dared her to go down the ravine under the bridge and, along with Grace, left her there in the snow after she had fallen through the ice.

When a theme recurs in fable, myth, and legend and in classical and modern literature, as does the theme of betrayal, it is clearly important. That is an understatement. Its importance is apparently in that it has meaning for us all. We have experienced it and have either a conscious or an unconscious memory of some great *let-down.* When *A Passage to India,* along with its other literary merits, touches on this deep knowledge, it becomes a classic. The knowledge is of universal significance, as are the legends and stories occurring in all languages and the symbolism consistent in various bodily and spiritual images, such as the number three: the third party; "thou shalt deny me thrice"; "Thrice hath Calphurnia in her sleep cried out, 'Help, ho! They murder Caesar'"; and the physical or mental wound—divorce court officers have told me how often they hear the word *wounded.* Portia, in attempting to persuade Brutus to trust her, says,

> *"I have made strong proof of my constancy*
> *Giving myself a voluntary wound*
> *Here in my thigh. Can I bear that with patience*
> *And not my husband's secrets?"*
>
> [Shakespeare, "Julius Caesar"]

The theme has an archetypal quality. In expounding his theory of archetypes, Jung described them as "inborn modes" —active, living dispositions that influence thought, feeling, and action, correlates of instinct. He writes:

> The inborn mode of acting has long been known as *instinct,* and for the inborn mode of psychic apprehension I have proposed the term *archetype.* Just as conscious apprehension gives our actions form and direction, so unconscious apprehension through the archetypes determines the form and direction of instinct. [Jung, 1921]

Jung was referring to a biological entity—a self-activating organism, "endowed with generative power", perhaps not dissimilar to the "innate releasing mechanism" postulated by Tinbergen, or the blueprint suggested by Bowlby when discussing the perception of pattern:

> In all such cases, we must suppose the individual organism has a copy of that pattern in its central nervous system and is structured to react in special kinds of way when it perceives a matching pattern in the environment and in other

kinds of way when it perceives no such patterns. [Bowlby, 1969]

To put the definition back into Jung's words, he referred to the

imprint which has arisen through the condensation of countless processes of a similar kind. . . . In this sense it is a precipitate, a typical basic form, of certain ever recurring psychic experiences. [Jung, 1921]

He also called the archetypes "primordial images". By "image" he did not mean the reflection of an external object but, rather, a fantasy only indirectly related to the reality of the external world.

I call the image primordial, when it possesses an archaic character and is in striking accord with familiar mythological motifs. [Jung, 1921]

Presumably the first felt betrayal of those who have been relatively well mothered in the first months of life is experienced during the weaning process—the end of an illusion of fusion and perfect mutuality. Perhaps "good-enough mothering" (Winnicott's term) in this early stage is about meeting the baby's illusion of omnipotence and protecting him from his own treachery when his hunger discomfort or anger may threaten to overpower him. But the illusion of fusion, of perfect understanding, of an ideal other who will never let one down has to be given up. The good-enough parent has to disillusion. To the innocent, this is treachery. It helps no child to be told, "This hurts me more than you". If the betrayal is to be creative, the betrayed needs support through acknowledgement of the hurt while he picks himself up and takes himself forward with his own interpretation of what has happened. That so many of the stories of betrayal concern brothers suggests that the birth of the next baby is also experienced as a betrayal of the parents' love.

We are speaking of the necessity of betrayal. Many of our most disturbed patients, however, have been, or have felt themselves to have been, betrayed too soon and too severely. Subsequent betrayals touch on these early wounds, and the response, fired by deep and early hurt, is primitive. Perhaps one important hallmark of maturity, of experience having gained ascendancy over innocence, is the ability to judge whom to trust and when and in which situation, and then to take the risk. In accordance with Jung's "principle of opposition" (Jung, 1917), there can be no trust without the possibility of betrayal, and there can be no betrayal if there has been no previous trust. We are not betrayed by our enemies; we are betrayed only by our friends, allies, intimates, and our nearest and dearest. It was only after Samson told Delilah "all his heart" that her betrayal of him to the Philistines was effective. On her previous attempts, he had failed to tell her where his "great strength lieth". The greater the love, loyalty, involvement, and commitment, the greater the sense of betrayal when it is felt that the trust is abused. As Hillman (1964) has said, "The critical moment of the great let down is when one is crucified by one's own trust". Or, more eloquently, Shakespeare wrote,

> "For Brutus, as you know, was Caesar's angel.
> Judge, O you Gods, how dearly Caesar loved him!
> This was the most unkindest cut of all;
> For when the noble Caesar saw him stab
> . . . Then burst his mighty heart."
>
> [Shakespeare, "Julius Caesar"]

And, as was told in Psalm 55:

> "It was not an enemy that reviled me
> or I might have borne it:
> it was not my foe that dealt so insolently with me
> or I might have hidden myself from him;
> but it was you a man like myself:
> my companion and my familiar friend."

A patient of mine well illustrated this point, that trust is the forerunner of betrayal.

My patient and her partner had both been promiscuous before they met. They were amazed that, in contrast to previous sexual relationships in which a grand passion had always dwindled from its early height, their love had grown slowly from an early liking. It had been an entirely different experience. She was thrilled when one of her dreams confirmed her newly emerging ability to depend on and trust her partner. A few days later she was very upset after what she called "a few bad days" for them. "After that dream", she said, "I felt quite betrayed. I do not think that is too strong a word." The "few bad days" occurred just before they were having to separate for some weeks—the first separation they had had to handle since they started living together. Trust had come into their lives, but so had the possibility of betrayal—sexual infidelity, even total abandonment. Could they sustain their new love through the enforced separation? Clearly, both of them had become quite anxious about this.

Just because of the preceding trust, another characteristic of betrayal is that it comes without expectation. If expected, it normally feels less treacherous. However, people who have experienced gross betrayal in early life and been left with little ability to trust may well spend much of their later life falling into situations of dubious trust, as if this is necessarily part of the "expected environment" (Hartman, 1958). Negative as this may sound, it also contains the seeds of hope. If they can discover that betrayal is not inevitable, some healing of the original wound takes place. An "old ghost" can be laid to rest.

However, many of those who have been severely betrayed when young are often the betrayers when older. They have learnt little about trust. In *Cat's Eye*, Elaine, at last able to move out of the role of victim of Cordelia, who "made me believe I was nothing", found that she had "a denser, more malevolent little triumph to finger; energy has passed between us and I am stronger. . . . The person I use my mean mouth on most is Cordelia. She doesn't even have to provoke me, I just use her as target practice."

Those who betray so often get themselves betrayed. The moral of the fable, "The Ass, the Fox and the Lion", is: "Betray a friend, and you'll often find you have ruined yourself."

Revenge (with a capital R) is one of the commonest of the primitive reactions to betrayal. The talion law—an eye for an eye and a tooth for a tooth—comes into operation. Welfare workers in Conciliation Services know well of the attempts to settle old scores (the longer this goes on, the meaner and pettier it so often becomes). Again, this is not just as negative as it sounds. Elaine had wanted Cordelia as a close friend. When words fail, one way of trying to get closer to another person is to get them to feel as one has felt oneself: "if he or she knows that feeling too, he will understand what it is like to be me. So I will get her to feel it as I do." In her turn, Cordelia had felt totally betrayed by her father. "She's frightened of not pleasing him. And yet he is not pleased. I've seen it many times, her dithering, fumble-footed efforts to appease him. But nothing she can ever do or say will ever be enough, because she is somehow the wrong person." (With two older sisters, we may guess she was not the much-longed-for boy.) In *A Passage to India*, Mrs Moore abandoned Adela and Dr Aziz only after she had felt totally abandoned: "If you don't know, you don't know."

Cynicism is another response. This denies the value of the previous love and trust. *All* love becomes a cheat, a trap, or a fraud. What has gone before is devalued. In the fable of "The Fox and the Grapes", the fox, having failed to reach the fine bunches of grapes, walks off with an air of dignity and unconcern, remarking, "I thought those grapes were ripe, but I see now they are quite sour". With this behaviour, however, the denial of the value of the past experience results in the betrayal of the self.

Forgiveness can be the sequel of betrayal. The big question for one ancient Abbot in his constant, obsessive musings was whether God had pardoned Judas or condemned him to everlasting hell.

The problem of forgiveness is that one is not really forgiving, if one can forgive easily; hurt or wound does not allow ease, and with no hurt there has been no betrayal. Forgiveness bereft of emotion remains a meaningless term. One cannot forgive to order, to the command to "think positively", or because one *should*. The word only becomes meaningful when the act is felt initially to be impossible. One step that has to be taken in the often long-fought-out inner conflict is that of daring to trust again, knowing that inevitably there is risk of further betrayal.

Forgiveness is harder for the betrayed when the betrayer is not carrying his own guilt and is attempting to unload it on others. If one party is to forgive, the other needs to atone. If unable to admit guilt, or attempting only to forget the deed, there is no atonement. As Hillman (1964) said, "a paradox of betrayal is the fidelity which both betrayed and betrayer keep, after the event, to its bitterness". Only within the environment of the bitterness created can the atonement have any reality. Once the bitterness and guilt are openly faced, they can recede, but the memory remains.

The degree to which people feel betrayed by their marriage partner depends not only on their continued involvement, but also on the covenant and troth, spoken and unspoken, that the couple made and gave in the first place. When attempting to understand people's behaviour when they feel betrayed, we need to take account of the idealization of the in-love state and the weight of expectation in the conscious and unconscious hopes vested in the partner. In seeking to promote the realization of his human nature, the individual attempts to correct earlier unsatisfactory experiences in later life events. In doing so, he gives himself a chance of healing old wounds. As I have suggested in other writings (Clulow & Mattinson, 1989; Mattinson, 1988), the seemingly fateful choice of one marriage partner rather than another contains the unconscious recognition and hope that this person can provide an environment in which there is the possibility of old fears being contained or even banished.

For those who have been severely betrayed in childhood, the possibility of further betrayal is one of the most salient fears. When another betrayal occurs, the old wounds are re-opened, and these will need as much attention from the therapist as the recent infidelity, abandonment, or whatever it is that feels so treacherous.

> One patient had found in adulthood, both with his wife and in his work, some salvation from treachery experienced early in his life. When he was a child, his father had "rubbished" him and rarely allowed him to do anything for himself. "That's a load of rubbish. You're not doing it properly. . . . Let me do it." His mother had always removed him from the scene and taken him shopping. He remained very dependent on her until, most sensibly, he married a dependable woman who, mildly agoraphobic, was always at home when he needed her. However, she behaved in a different way from his father and mother in that she said, "We can do it", and "You can do it". He no longer felt rubbished. Under her tutelage he claimed his own strength and became a competent person, particularly

when he was given the space to be precise and orderly. It was as if he needed order and predictability to keep the inner rubbish at bay. His job as an Apron Manager at an international airport required his precision. He parked aeroplanes immaculately, and he vividly described the "snarl-up" if planes were out of position. Although jeered at by colleagues for his pedantic ways, he had a boss who respected his methods and did not interfere with his parking plans.

This patient became depressed when he acquired a new boss, a much younger man who over-ruled his parking arrangements. Again he felt rubbished. His depression deepened when he was offered redundancy. Coinciding with this, he could no longer be sure of his wife when she was taken ill and had to go into hospital. All his terrors were revived, and again he felt totally betrayed.

As therapists, we need to be aware that when a breach of trust has been of immense significance in the childhood of the patient, betrayal and one of its negative sequels may well come to be enacted in the therapeutic encounter. If we find that we have deserted our normally reliable stance and that it is one patient rather than another that we have let down—inadvertently, as it may have seemed at the time—we need to understand not only more about the wounds we have re-opened but, even more important, the unconscious pressure we have been subjected to in getting us to re-play the scenario.

One patient was very restrained and wary when she first met her therapist. She responded with a smile when he suggested she might be afraid that he would look down on her and that she was not worth his taking any trouble. She was then able to use the time and describe the quandary she was in, but she queried the trustworthiness of the therapist when she said, "Nowhere is confidential".

The following week the therapist had influenza, but he wrote to her and explained why he could not keep the second appointment they had arranged. She answered this letter, but she declined any further contact: "I hope you are feeling better. . . . I hope you don't think too bad of me if I cancel the appointment you suggested." Because of her initial hesitancy, the therapist wrote again and offered another session, but on the appointed day he failed to check with reception when he was not notified of her arrival. Something in this patient's approach to the therapist was diffident enough to get her to be the one who was forgotten. Forgotten patients are not just the fault of an otherwise reliable receptionist. If the patient had been less ambivalent about trusting the therapist, she could have reminded the receptionist of her presence instead of sitting in the waiting room for 40 minutes. When she was eventually discovered, she showed in the 20 minutes left of the therapist's available time that she had, in fact, made good use of the previous interview. Another appointment was made, but, not surprisingly, she chose to cancel it and was not seen again.

If the patient can be held, the old wounds, now bleeding in the therapy, are at hand and available for therapeutic work. We may be made to experience what the patient has previously felt and currently feels. We may well experience a stab in the back and our confidence draining away when the patient starts to deny any value of the previous months' or years' work or launches into a retaliatory attack on our inadequacy. The anger that is released in respect of our untrustworthiness may be intensified by the suppressed anger initially felt by a powerless child at the time the initial treachery—neglect, desertion, or abuse—took place. Therapists, perhaps previously idealized and now fallen from grace, will need to acknowledge and take full responsibility for their contribution towards the bitterness before forgiveness can occur. He or she will need to be forgiven before forgiveness can take place in the marriage.

It is also important to remind ourselves that, as therapists, we should never offer a Garden of Eden, as some patients will try to force us to do. As long as we can acknowledge and regret them, our mistakes—assuming they are not felt to be the ultimate stab in the back—may well be an important factor in our patients giving up some of their innocence in favour of a more realistic trust.

A THERAPEUTIC APPROACH TO THE COUPLE RELATIONSHIP

Freud has postulated the process of *working through* as an essential part of the psychoanalytic procedure. To put it in a nutshell, this means enabling the patient to experience his emotions, anxieties, and past situations over and over again both in relation to the analyst and to different people and situations in the patient's present and past life.

Melanie Klein

A THERAPEUTIC APPROACH
TO THE COUPLE RELATIONSHIP

INTRODUCTION

All the chapters in this volume have included discussion of clinical material, primarily to illustrate the main theoretical themes being presented. It has already been said that the development of psychoanalysis and psychotherapeutic practice involves the constant interweaving of theory and clinical technique: theory informs clinical practice, and limitations discovered in clinical work may result in the subsequent evolution of theory. In relation to couple psychotherapy, object relations theory in particular has substantially influenced the development of a theoretical understanding of intimate couple interaction and has also influenced the nature of psychotherapeutic work with couples. Though couple psychotherapy draws on psychoanalytic theory and practice and applies it to the intrapsychic and interpersonal system of the couple, it has also developed a theory and practice particular to an understanding of and working with couples.

The two final chapters focus primarily on technical and clinical issues, though inevitably theoretical issues are also discussed. Both are written from the point of view of clinical work with couples using two therapists, working either conjointly or in parallel therapist–partner sessions. This is often, though by no means always, the practice in the TIMS, and it could be argued that for some couples this would be the psychotherapeutic intervention that is most appropriate to their need. The nature of the projective system operating between the couple may offer some diagnostic indication as to whether one or two therapists may be most appropriately employed (Ruszczynski, 1992).

However, whether one or two therapists are working with a couple, the primary focus of interest remains the shared conscious and unconscious images of relating and interaction that the patient couple bring into the therapeutic encounter and that will be transferred into the relationships in the consulting room. Internal unconscious object relations will determine the nature of external relationships.

Alison Lyons, in "Therapeutic Intervention in Relation to the Institution of Marriage" (chapter ten), takes up some central clinical issues. She suggests that the setting of the couple psychotherapy, which includes the therapist(s), offers the couple a "breathing space" within which reflection and self-realization may be possible. She stresses the point that internal images stemming from each partner's experiences of their parents' marriages and their relationship to the parental marriage will influence the way in which the partners make use of both each other in their intimate relationship, and the psychotherapist(s) in the course of the couple psychotherapy.

Alison Lyons goes on to discuss the rationale for seeing couples either together in conjoint sessions, separately with each partner having their own therapist, or with one therapist seeing the couple together. She illustrates this by giving two clinical examples, which demonstrate some of the diagnostic differences revealed in the initial assessments that led to one couple being seen mostly in conjoint meetings with two therapists, and another couple, who were never seen together but only in parallel individual sessions with their own therapist.

In "Thinking About and Working With Couples" (chapter eleven), I give a final overview of some of the central themes in the theory and practice of psychotherapy with couples. The chapter briefly outlines object relations theory, particularly as it has been influenced by some of the concepts introduced by Klein and her colleagues, and shows how it is a particularly appropriate construct with which to think about the intimate couple relationship. Many of the themes discussed in the earlier chapters are gathered into this one.

The core theoretical concept is that of unconscious partner choice, based on mutual projective and introjective identification, which offers the possibility of both developmental and defensive containment. *The relationship **itself**, alongside the internal capacities of the two partners, offers an arena for growth and development.* The degree to which this potential of the couple relationship is fulfilled depends on the nature of the shared anxieties and shared defences of the couple (their internal object relations) and on the vicissitudes of living with which all couples have to deal during the course of their shared life.

The second part of this chapter discusses the clinical understanding and use of transference and countertransference in psychotherapeutic work with couples. The major differences between individual psychoanalytic psychotherapy and psychotherapy with couples is that the couple in psychotherapy will bring into the consulting room their own "transference" and "countertransference" to each other. During the course of the couple psychotherapy, this real, meaningful, and powerful relationship, both in the consulting room and in the on-going life of the couple, will exist alongside and interweave with the transference and countertransference that will develop in the relationship to the therapist(s). Therefore, there may be said to be at least *two* transference–countertransference arenas that give access to a therapeutic understanding of internal object relations and how these internal images influence external relationships (Ruszczynski, 1992).

Both of these more specifically clinical chapters start from the point that has been stressed in all the previous chapters: the institution of the couple relationship offers a vehicle for psychological containment and development. If this capacity falters or fails, some couples may choose to seek psychotherapeutic help. The task of the couple psychotherapist is to provide a setting within which the couple may explore the nature of their internal object relations, as revealed in their "transference" to each other and in their transference to the therapist(s), with a view to restoring, if possible, the capacity of their relationship to go on providing the therapeutic possibilities inherent in intimate attachment.

CHAPTER TEN

Therapeutic intervention in relation to the institution of marriage

Alison Lyons

I t is questionable whether monogamous marriage provides either the most practical and comfortable or the easiest way in which to live and to rear children. Its limitations and inherent frustrations are obvious. The case against it has always been a strong one. Its developmental function is equally obvious, but as this can also be seen to serve destructive purposes, the case against it is strengthened. Marriage partners do stifle as well as sustain each other and can, in turn, stultify as well as nourish their children.

However, as those cultures practising monogamous marriage have been, to date, the most successful at surviving, it would seem that marriage as an institution has an evolutionary value and is worth a pause for consideration before it is labelled as an anachronism in post-industrial society.

Long-term commitments, it has been suggested, are no longer in tune with the needs of technological advance; and marriage in the future should be envisaged as a "throw-away" relationship. The propositions to be examined in this chapter are (1) that as an institution, monogamous marriage has certain attributes that give it a unique value as the cradle for psychic development, and (2) that this value can be enhanced by conscious effort to improve the quality of marriage. These propositions will finally be explored in relation to two couples who came for help to the Institute of Marital Studies. (At the time of writing—1973—the Tavistock Institute of Marital Studies was known by its previous name, the Institute of Marital Studies. See chapter one.)

Considered as a unit in the series of institutions to which an individual can commit himself during his life, marriage may be distinguished by the many-sided, even paradoxical, nature of the commitment it demands. The entrance levy of added responsibilities and legally enforceable obligations at once confers a hall-mark of maturity. The couple are congratulated on their success. But the rejoicing, as they declare their commitment and publicly display the nature of its possibilities and limitations—each other—to their relatives and friends, is not solely in honour of a maturational step. It is also an acknowledgement of the right to regress. The couple have acquired in each other a framework in which they can relax, make love, and enjoy baby-talk.

This opportunity for regression may or may not eventually prove to have been in the service of each one's personal development, but for the moment it will be regarded as if it were so. Provided the couple meet their new obligations, pay the rent, and care for the garden, no one is going to find it regrettable if, in their newly found attachment, the young marrieds cannot bear to be out of one another's sight. And, if the neighbours are amused at the clinging on the front door step, they will also be touched, and may even feel sad, to realize how soon this phase of re-enacted attachment behaviour will give way to a state when a perfunctory wave will do. No one will find their behaviour pathological nor dream of suggesting that the couple should "pull themselves together and snap out of it".

At the outset, therefore, and precisely because of its inherent paradox—its promise of freedom within a framework of constraint—this institution can be seen to offer each individual the opportunity to achieve real emotional growth as distinct from its instantly acquired hall-mark. The extent to which this opportunity can be grasped will, however, depend upon the capacity for physical and psychological interaction that each individual brings from the light of his past experience into the relationship. Paramount factors in this past experience will be the degree of security with which the parental attachments of each partner were originally established and the consequent ease or difficulty with which an attachment to a new figure can be made. These considerations affecting the degree to which developmental possibilities available in any particular marriage can be exploited also hold good for therapeutic partnerships and are the factors that will be more specifically explored in relation to the couples to be described later.

Bowlby has drawn attention to the fact that an infant's experience of how his parents maintain, or fail to maintain, their relationship with him plays a vital part in the way he will later organize his own relationships (Bowlby, 1973b). One cannot escape the conclusion from clinical work that the child also experiences and internalizes the parents' way of relating each to the other.

At the Institute of Marital Studies we find ourselves confronted by couples whose means of maintaining their relationships will include a variety of unconscious agreements. This kind of mutual dependency is a quite normal part of any marriage; but when it imposes too heavy a limitation on the partner's independent action and autonomy, then the price has become too high. In other words, the price for these unconscious agreements designed to make an uncertain world seem more certain than it actually is has become that of finding it less satisfying than it need actually be. This kind of interplay can also be seen as the couple's unconsciously determined method of maintaining their sense of closeness and of being held by one another. Our therapeutic intention is, therefore, to provide a situation in which our understanding of this process can be communicated to the couple in a way that will give both a feeling of being held through a necessary period of flux and will allow them to have a more reflective, less defensive perception of themselves, each other, and their children.

The therapeutic technique through which the staff at the Institute of Marital Studies attempt to communicate this understanding to the couples who come to them may be based on either two-person meetings, where each of the married pair has an individual therapist, three-person meetings, where there is one therapist with a married pair, or four-person meetings of two therapists with a married pair. It therefore becomes relevant to consider the rationale behind these various ways of intervening.

Skynner (1969) has outlined some indications and contra-indications for conjoint and for individually based forms of family therapy. Dicks (1967) writes authoritatively on the use of both forms of therapy in hospital work. There now seems little disagreement among practitioners about the particular usefulness of conjoint therapy for couples who are both functioning at a basically part-object or undifferentiated level with the concomitantly extensive use of such primitive defence mechanisms as denial and splitting. This agreement is based on the fact that in such families there is a sense in which, to use Skynner's words: "No true individual as yet exists" (Skynner, 1969).

Opinions, however, differ on the contra-indications for conjoint therapy. Clinical observations by the staff at the Institute of Marital Studies suggest that when married partners have begun to see and feel worried and sad about what each one is doing to the other in their relationship, then the couple need individual help to bear this painful guilt. Individuals who are at this level of development are struggling to acknowledge the coexistence, in others as well as themselves, of destructive and creative impulses and to sustain, with the necessary discretion, the moral conflicts that such acknowledgement requires. This would accord with Skynner's suggestion that for couples who have reached but not yet integrated the depressive position conjoint therapy is unsuitable. Later, when the individuals can more easily bear their awareness of guilt and separateness, then either conjoint or individual therapy seems to be equally appropriate.

The different therapeutic needs of the two couples now to be discussed were revealed in their intake interviews and led us to adopt different techniques for each of them. As a result, one couple, the Bankses, have often been seen conjointly, whereas the other couple, the Thomases, never have. Conjoint meetings here refer to four-person sessions. Each of the married pair has an individual therapist. Conjoint meetings apart, the most important difference between marital therapy as practised at the Institute and other forms of individual therapy is the understanding, explicit from the outset, that the bond of confidentiality between therapist and patient does not include communication between the therapeutic pair, who, on the contrary, not only have the same freedom of discussion as that enjoyed by the married pair but regard it as part of their technique to discuss the content of the therapeutic sessions between themselves. Unlike the married pair, however, the therapeutic pair are bound in confidence against divulging to their respective patients anything disclosed to them by the fellow therapist. The importance of this structure will be clear in the light of the previously discussed rationale for variations in technique.

From a statistical point of view it would seem surprising that these two couples had such differing therapeutic needs. From a superficial glance they appear amazingly similar. Both couples are in their late thirties, have been married for nine years, and have been working with us for the past eighteen months. Each couple has two boys, one of school and one of pre-school age. It also happens that both husbands follow professions that entail a certain amount of travelling, and both wives follow independent but home-based professions. All four people are in familiar contact with the psychoanalytic world. Both couples were referred with rather pressing urgency by their medical advisers, who feared for the vulnerability of the children.

In each case the couple's initial enthusiasm for "the Tavistock" rather quickly gave way to complaints about our geographic and temporal inflexibility, culminating in an outburst against "the administration" even before therapy itself had started. The fact that neither of these couples could pursue their exploration of the Tavistock's therapeutic possibilities without being very perturbed by minor frustration suggests that as institutions their marriages could not at the time of referral sustain the tensions necessary to promote growth. As it turns out, however, one pair of these apparently evenly matched couples, the Thomases, has, in fact, been able to use their therapy to create a much safer, livelier, and more enjoyable climate between them, and they have acquired a greater degree of individual freedom in the process; whereas the other pair, the Bankses, are still having to battle it out in an extremely painful way between themselves and with their therapists, with the outcome still in some doubt.

As well as being matched for age, duration of marriage, sex and number of children, education, and socio-economic status, these two couples also presented their problems in similar terms. The heart of the matter was in each case an inability to feel safe together. None of the four people involved had a really well-established sexual image of him or herself, and both couples felt that their marriages were in danger of breaking up.

So much for the similarities—which on paper were so striking. The differences, which immediately became apparent in their intake interviews, lay in the level of their unconscious defence systems. The couple for whom the outcome of therapy remains in doubt predominantly employs the most primitive defence systems—denial and splitting. Each partner blames the other and each thinks the other "mad". Sexual life is kept in a separate compartment, secret and "good". Children have to be seen to be and kept "undamaged". Fundamentally, each partner feels the other is impossible to live with.

Mr and Mrs Thomas did not blame each other. They were both extremely aware of and almost over-concerned about the effect of their difficulties on the children. They felt that their sexual relationship left much to be desired and that it reflected their general unease together. Each was concerned about his and her own psychopathological contribution to joint problems, and both were anxious to find a more satisfying and benign way of functioning together. Their defences were mainly intellectualization and the typical depressive mechanism of turning against the self.

Further exploration with both these couples revealed that their contrasting control systems, if not originally based on, were nevertheless unconsciously reinforced by experiences of parental interaction of a highly significant kind. Mr and Mrs Banks had each experienced a parental marriage that failed, and Mr and Mrs Thomas had each experienced a parental marriage that had at least succeeded in maintaining a relationship. At this level the only similarity between these four people is the shared parental image of a father who was "absent" in the sense that he did not offer the mother an emotional security that might have enabled her to support her children's gradual moves towards autonomy. Although there was no divorce, both the parental families of Mr and Mrs Banks were physically separated while the Bankses were children. All four parents are still alive and still live apart.

For Mr and Mrs Thomas, father's absence was, in each case, emotional. Physically the parental families remained intact throughout childhood. Furthermore, Mrs Thomas' mother —the only surviving parent—remains aloof. In so doing, she exacerbates her daughter's rivalry with her brother, but at the same time she has given Mrs Thomas a chance to work through her feelings of rejection and then, from the security of her new therapeutic attachment, to move towards autonomy. During a recent holiday, a set-to occurred which showed the way this movement is being exercised and reinforced by Mrs Thomas in an attempt to find what she feels to be the appropriate "distance" between herself and her mother. At the risk of forfeiting her mother's company to her more accommodating brother, she was able to stand firm about the dates that she and her husband could manage, and she did not give way under the combined pressure of mother and brother as she might previously have done.

This process of distancing has been far more difficult for the Bankses, whose parents help to keep the earlier psychic situation brewing by remaining in continuous and disturbing contact with their children. Mr Banks's mother, for instance, expects to be contacted every day.

For the Bankses, the break-up of their parents' marriages seems to have left in each of them a quality of instability that emerges all too clearly in their own marriage. They spend most of their time together quarrelling. Mr Banks uses his professional commitments to leave his wife and family from time to time, although he can never leave them entirely, despite his conscious dissatisfactions. If one looks beneath the surface, their quarrels appear to be conducted in the hope that each partner will magically change and, in so doing, preserve the fantasy of an ideal partnership. In fact, neither partner has attained that level of psychic functioning which would at times permit postponement of the satisfaction of his or her own need in favour of the other's—a manifestation of the depressive position in which turning against the self is actually valuable. Each constantly demands from the other more than it is psychologically possible for him or her to give. Their attempted solutions to their problems by means of denial and splitting are regressive rather than developmental.

The core of the therapeutic difficulty encountered has been how to enable either Mr or Mrs Banks to see the difference between their present interaction and the stereotypes they have internalized. That is, although each one can, at times, manage to postpone satisfaction of a need in favour of the other, the other can always be relied on to fail to perceive this. This unconscious collusion to keep the *status quo* springs from their joint fears. They are afraid, on the one hand, of acknowledging closeness or the tenderness that threatens to dissolve boundaries and leave each in the imagined danger of being totally swallowed up by the other and, on the other hand, of a separateness that is equally complete. These two people have no experience of being alone and yet together.

Administrative chance led to a further difference in therapeutic structure between these couples. The Bankses each have a therapist of the same sex as themselves, whereas the Thomases both have women therapists. The fact that a couple functioning like the Bankses, with their impaired ability to symbolize, were each able to work in individual sessions with therapists of the same sex as themselves as well as conjointly is a lucky accident that our therapeutic resources would not necessarily be able to repeat. The importance to Mr Banks in particular of a chance to experience in relation to his male therapist a positive homosexual bond can be understood when it is known that Mr Thomas and Mr Banks both had the shared experience of sleeping in their parents' bedroom. But, while Mr Thomas continued to do so until he was nineteen, his father remained a part of the scene. Mr Banks' father, on the other hand, had quit the scene when his son was eleven years old, leaving him exposed to the full impact of his mother's presence in the one bedroom of their new home. It is not surprising that the closeness of the marriage served as a severe test to the precariously established autonomy of both these husbands, nor that Mr Banks's efforts to maintain it should force him to leave home from time to time and to maintain at home a degree of distance through constant quarrelling.

Mr Thomas's struggle for autonomy, although arduous, had not been so traumatically curtailed. Despite the disturbing atmosphere at home, he had had sufficient emotional breathing space in which to develop reflective processes and could, therefore, contain his flight from the threatening closeness in fantasy, without having to act it out in reality. This ability to symbolize also meant that he could find buried feelings for his father reactivated in relation to a woman therapist.

When Mr Thomas came into therapy, he was, in fact, obsessed with guilty, frightening, and exciting sexual thoughts that were direct legacies from the stimulating but repressive experiences at his mother's side in the parental bedroom. As these experiences were gradually worked through in the course of therapy, he found that he could afford to maintain a more prolonged and consciously committed contact with his wife. Meanwhile, her interlocking defences of frigidity and failure to acknowledge her husband's potency also gave way in response to her therapist's and later her husband's more positive approach.

Mr Thomas's most telling experience of his parents' interaction did not in fact take place in their bedroom. It took place in the living room when his father returned from the family business with the weekly takings. The money was poured on the floor at mother's feet, and an excited counting then took place between the parents, which was the high spot of the week.

Mr Thomas began to realize that, in identifying with this form of parental intercourse, similar countings and recountings took place between himself and his mother in which he would relate his exploits and to which she responded in excitement and a tacit agreement to leave father out. It was irritating for Mr Thomas to perceive the relatively unmoved acceptance accorded to similar fantasies by his therapist—me—and to give up the guilty, conspiratorial excitement that these evoked in him. For a long time he did his best to get a livelier response and finally produced his first recollected step towards autonomy. When aged three, he bravely asserted to his mother's back that he wished he had a younger and prettier mother—someone like Aunt Margaret. We were both aware by this time of the significance to him of his wife's much younger therapist who is also called Margaret. When the tears and recriminations did not follow, as mother's had, he was able to accept my interpretation of this unconscious attempt to get the desired though feared but repressive behaviour, from which there was no authoritative father to turn to for support.

Such impulses have been more easily and quickly neutralized in the course of therapy than one might expect from general experience of individual therapy; being marital work, however, it was less unexpected because of the new possibilities for physical excitement and pleasure that were developing in the marriage. Mrs Thomas had in fact a similar image of parental intercourse in that for her parents the "high spot" of the month took place when the account books for the family business were checked between them. Father's generous recognition of mother's expertise in this activity was almost the only remembered evidence of his admiration that Mrs Thomas carried with her into her marriage, and she found it very difficult to give up her own "expert professional" response which her husband valued highly but could also be hurt by, in favour of a more feeling response that could include a recognition of her own desire for love and attachment. This, of course, became easier as his responses became more trustworthy. In a recent holiday break he was able to support her in her efforts to achieve the more appropriate distance, already referred to, between herself and her mother.

During the course of therapy Mr Thomas gradually severed himself from the suffocating aspects of his mother's memory, and this severance became symbolized for him in a new-found ability to "let go" physically in many hitherto restricted activities such as swimming, dancing, and music-making. It was as though he had begun to take for his own the famous words of Kierkegaard: "Only that part of the past is worth remembering which can become the present."

Benign recollection can, however, only occur if there has been something benign to recollect. There can be no doubt that Mr Thomas's earliest experiences with his mother had given him enough unconscious memories of a safe closeness on which he could rely when the time eventually came for him to "let go". Where the earliest experiences have been mainly persecutory, the task of helping people to detach themselves from these bad memories is much more formidable, as is the case with Mr and Mrs Banks. Like that part of the past which is being unconsciously relived in the transference, the strain on the therapists will vary with the degree to which the patient's capacity to symbolize has been impaired. It has never been difficult for me to remain relatively unmoved and unafraid of the fantasies that so frightened Mr Thomas, because I knew that, even when he was feeling angry with me for the lack of excitement in my response, he was also relieved and would be ready to relinquish his hope of a gratifying re-enactment of childhood triumphs in favour of symbolic exploration. This was not true of the Bankses. Although they are both well-educated and articulate people, words would not serve them to communicate the quality of the anxiety that engulfed them both. This had to be communicated to each other and to their therapists by imposing the sort of suspense that they themselves endured. No one had ever to know what anyone was going to do next, and everyone had to live under the continual threat of disaster. When the major part of the communication received by therapists has to be at this level, then their ability to allow themselves to become disturbed by it and then to explore the disturbance symbolically becomes a most important, but arduous, part of the therapy.

Mrs Banks could take her therapist's peaceful acceptance of her emotions as something good in contra-distinction to the way in which her feelings were and are still exploited by both parents. But there are very few peaceful experiences to put in the place of the sexual excitement that the parents' fighting had engendered.

If something "good" happens to the Bankses, they cannot bear it. They don't know themselves. In fact, this couple look physically ill when things are better between them. But as soon as the quarrelling starts again, they pick up and seem much fitter. Anything "good" from therapy is intensely alarming because of its threat to the *status quo*, so that whenever they come to a "foursome" after a peaceful period it is predictable that they will—to quote a favourite expression of theirs—"knock the living daylights" out of their therapists.

However, between them, the therapists have held on to their seat belts and to their belief in the possibility of development. Something of this does seem to have been transferred to the couple and is expressed by them in a very concrete way—that is, they have at last been able to choose a more suitable house in which to live.

But whether the development can ever be internalized remains an open question. A hopeful sign may be that for the first time recently Mrs Banks has talked of one of the children having a problem. This suggests that the splitting on which this couple has depended may not be as total as it has seemed to be in the past. If this is so, their children—the next generation—will be relieved of some of the pressure on them to remain the perceptually good, undamaged objects through whom their parents are kept alive and together.

To sum up: in the course of their development children will normally select and internalize certain features of their parents' personalities and means of adaptation, until they have gradually acquired a more or less stable self-image. Any environment that cannot afford sufficient shelter from anxiety will preclude this normal process of selectivity, and the child may then have to resort to the pathological solution of swallowing his parents whole. The resulting tie to an unreal, idealized, or totally denigrated image of the parental marriage has eventually to be realized and consciously explored if it is ever to be relinquished in favour of a more adequate system. A good-enough marriage can provide the framework within which the lost "breathing space" can be found. It can afford unanxious time for reflection—time in which to become aware of and express hitherto repressed fears and wishes, to try them out and discover that the dread consequences do not ensue. The intimacy of marriage, in which the closeness to another person can support, although it may also threaten, established autonomy as well as further the development of a separate identity, is necessarily reminiscent of the infant's earliest attachment to his mother. At the same time, it need not lead to an exact repetition of the pattern derived from that relationship. The capacity to symbolize brings with it the capacity to distinguish past from present and the ability to recognize and help to create a new emotional climate.

The majority of couples who come to the Institute of Marital Studies today not only recognize that marriage can serve this developmental function, they come demanding that it should. And in that sense they seem to be shouldering the task of trying to provide stability and continuity in an increasingly fluctuating environment.

CHAPTER ELEVEN

Thinking about
and working with couples

Stanley Ruszczynski

C entral to psychoanalytic psychotherapy with couples—
as with individual patients—is the view that human
behaviour is directed and governed by unconscious as
well as conscious motivation. In simple terms, the term "unconscious" is a description of that part of the mind that is outside
consciousness. More specifically, the word "unconscious" refers
to that layer of the mind which contains repressed thoughts,
feelings, needs, and wishes that cannot be allowed into consciousness, but which influence and affect behaviour and experience as much as, if not more than, conscious needs and
wishes.

This unconscious part of the mind is not passive: it is dynamic and seeks expression. It seeks another person who may
be able to meet or respond to these repressed needs and
wishes, not necessarily with any conscious awareness of having done so. As Freud said, "It is a very remarkable thing that
the unconscious of one human being can react upon that of
another without passing through the conscious . . . descrip-
tively speaking, the fact is incontestable" (Freud, 1915e).

In classical Freudian theory, this leads to instinct theory: an
understanding of human behaviour as primarily motivated and

driven by the need to have repressed wishes met, and hence gain pleasure, or at least to reduce the feelings of displeasure.

Through the work of Balint, Fairbairn, Winnicott, Klein, and Bion, the development of object relations theory made a subtle but profound shift in the understanding of human behaviour. From infant observation, the findings of child analysis, the greatly enriched data coming from clinical work particularly with psychotic patients, and the growing understanding and clinical use of transference and then countertransference, an interest developed in the primacy of the relationship between the new-born infant and his environment (Sutherland, 1963). This resulted in a move away from the one-person psychology of Freud's instinct theory towards an understanding of human behaviour as being motivated by a search for another person with whom one can relate. Object relations theory obliges us to stop thinking of the individual in isolation, but to see him in his interaction with others in the environment, both consciously and unconsciously.

Freud, of course, was not unaware of object relating, and the expression does arise in his writings (Freud, 1917e, 1931b). However, although the idea is inherent in his work, it does not play an overt part in his conceptual schema.

Since the 1930s, the notion of object relations has generally attained much importance, and today it constitutes a major theoretical parameter. It is a part of a movement of ideas not confined to psychology or psychoanalysis. In the physical sciences, too, the organism under investigation is now more often examined in the context of its surroundings (Laplanche & Pontalis, 1973). In the psychological field, we now have what we could call a person-to-person psychology, and this has led to such developments as family and group therapy, be it psychoanalytic or systemic; it has led to communications theory; and it underpins the increasing interest in the transference and countertransference inherent in any therapeutic encounter. The concepts of projective and introjective identification and container/contained (Bion, 1962b, 1967) add further depth to an understanding of object relating. This conceptual and clinical shift provides the bedrock upon which psychoanalytic psychotherapy with couples is based.

Interaction in object relating

In couple psychotherapy, the focus of clinical interest is the *interaction* between the two people who make up a relationship. The patient, as it were, may be said to be the relationship or marriage. There is nothing unique in this orientation. Bion, writing about how he personally worked with his individual analytic patients, says, "The relationship between two people is a two way affair and in so far as one is concerned with demonstrating that relationship, it is not a matter of talking about analyst and analysand; it is talking about something *between* the two of them" (Bion, 1978, italics added).

Symington, in an essay on psychoanalysis and truth, says that truth is not grasped in a moment of insight *within* an individual, but, rather, it is grasped in dialogue with another or others, "it emerges *in between*", he says (Symington, 1986). Contemporary Freudians refer to wish-fulfilment in object relations terms. For example, "the child who has a wish to cling to the mother has . . . a mental representation of himself clinging to the mother. But he also has . . . a mental representation of the mother responding to his clinging in a particular way . . ." (Sandler & Sandler, 1978). And Winnicott, of course, writes of the space between two people, initially that between mother and infant, which he sees as the arena for play, communication, creativity, and healthy living (Winnicott, 1971).

In a couple relationship, that which happens in the space between the two people is referred to as marital interaction. Marital interaction refers to the constant and necessary tension inherent in any human relationship—that is, the tension between, on the one hand, the autonomy and individuality of each partner, and, on the other hand, the partnership they aspire to. This conflict or tension may be played out in a number of ways: between independence and dependence, between self-assertion and sharing, between exploration and safety, and ultimately between love and hate. All of these conflicts stem from the earliest experiences of infancy. Some are consciously known about and managed in the couple relationship, but unconscious conflicts and tensions are *also* brought into a marriage, with an unconscious hope for resolution or satisfaction.

To explain this, I need to refer to another basic premise: that

> as we develop from infancy onwards we never completely
> forget the ways of functioning which we have learned ear-
> lier, and particularly the ways which we learned first of all
> as infants. Thus the most mature adult carries with him,
> quite unconsciously, ways of functioning and relating to
> people which are essentially infantile. To understand these
> ways we must return to the world of the infant. [Allingham,
> 1987]

What are these essentially infantile ways of functioning?
From the moment of birth, and indeed from even earlier, the
human infant is engaged in a struggle to reach his or her full
physical and psychological potential. At the very beginning this
struggle may appear to be primarily a biological one: the new-
born infant seems to be preoccupied with bodily needs. However, by the very fact of being in need of a caring, feeding
mother, the infant is involved in a relationship. As Winnicott
writes, "There is no such thing as an infant, meaning of course
that whenever one finds an infant one finds maternal care"
(Winnicott, 1975).

From the very beginning, the infant is a subject taking the
mother as his object of attachment. But the mother in her own
right is also a subject and takes the infant as her object of care
and concern. A complex interaction, therefore, goes on between
the two, and within that, adaptive and defensive processes of
each are geared in with those of the other and have to function
in relation to the other (Bannister & Pincus, 1965). The nature
of this first object relation becomes a prototype for all subsequent childhood and adult relationships.

The genesis of object relation theory is contained in Freud,
who wrote, "the character of the ego is a precipitate of abandoned object-cathexes and . . . it contains the history of these
object choices . . . the effects of the first identifications made in
earliest childhood will be general and lasting" (Freud, 1923b).

The process of growth and development, therefore, with its
pleasures and pains, satisfactions and conflicts, remains im-
printed on the individual's psychology. No infant will have all
of his needs met—mothers can only be good enough, to use

Winnicott's expression, and not perfect. Frustration is an inevitable part of the process of growth, and defences are built up to
manage failure and disappointment. Mechanisms of defence,
as ways of managing ourselves in the world and the world in
ourselves, become major determinants of our sense of ourselves and of our object relations.

It has been said that the term "object relations" is a "trou-
blesome term" (Greenberg & Mitchell, 1983). In its broadest
sense, the term "object relations theory", "refers to attempts
within psychoanalysis to . . . confront the potentially confound-
ing observation that people live simultaneously in an external
and an internal world. . . . The term thus designates theories,
or aspects of theories, concerned with exploring the relationship between real external people and internal images and
residues of relations with them" (Greenberg & Mitchell, 1983).

In their definition of the concept of "object relation",
Laplanche and Pontalis (1973) tell us that the word "object", in
this context, has to be understood in a particular way: the other
person in a relationship is described as an "object" in the sense
that unconscious needs, conflicts, wishes, and fears are directed at him, and these will determine the nature of the relationship just as much as, if not more than, the reality of that
other person. Object relations theory, therefore, is concerned
with the relations of the subject to his objects, *not* simply with
the relationship between the two, which is an interpersonal
relationship:

> It is not only the real relationship with others that deter-
> mines the subject's individual life, but *the specific way in
> which the subject apprehends his relationships with his ob-
> jects* (both internal and external). It always implies an un-
> conscious relationship to these objects. [Kohon, 1986, ital-
> ics added]

We are therefore talking of an *inter*-relating, of a fluid interaction between two people, both of whom are simultaneously
treating the other as object of their needs, wishes, and conflicts, conscious and unconscious. This holds true in every human relationship, even that of the mother and infant, where the
relationship is substantially shaped and limited by the radical
difference in their needs and capabilities.

A model of growth and development

A theory of object relations, as a model for understanding human relationships and the process of psychological growth and development, was substantially delineated by Melanie Klein, who paid particular attention to the internal and intra-psychic aspects of object relations. She posits two positions of mental development: the first, operative in the first few months of life, she calls the "paranoid–schizoid". The immature ego of the infant struggles from birth to manage the anxiety stirred up by the inborn polarity of the life and death instincts. It is also immediately exposed to the impact of external reality, which is loving, gentle, and life-giving or rejecting, cold, and anxiety-producing. The primitive defences used to deal with these conflictual experiences are splitting and projection, and thus the leading anxiety becomes paranoid. Other defences include denial, idealization, and, most important, projective identification.

These defence mechanisms, and especially that of projection, are the earliest determinants of the nature of primitive object relations. These are actually part-object relations, because at this stage the infant does not experience a whole object called a mother, for example, but, rather, a pair of hands, a face, a voice, or a breast. A legacy therefore is left which produces a tendency to project out parts of the self, bad and good, that are felt to be threatening or threatened. (Good parts, if felt to be threatened by internal bad objects, can be projected for safe-keeping.) This splitting and projection results in potential aspects of the self being repudiated or disowned. Hence they are lost to the person and inhibit the possibility of experiencing the full potential of the self and of relationships.

As the first months go by and the infant approaches the second half of the first year of life, powers of perception, conceptualization, and thinking are developing. This inherent maturational process combines with the actual experience of the containment provided by the good-enough mother, who is able to produce a preponderance of good feelings over bad. This gives strength to the good feelings and lessens the fear of the bad, and so reduces the amount of anxiety previously experienced. As a result, the good and bad feelings no longer have to be kept so separate, and so the infant's capacity to integrate experiences begins to grow.

The infant now moves into what Melanie Klein calls the "depressive position". The mother who feeds and satisfies is slowly recognized as the same mother who frustrates and deprives. The infant begins to realize that he both loves and hates the same person. This produces a fear that his hatred may damage the person whom he loves, and so he experiences concern and guilt.

The leading anxiety at this time, therefore, is depressive. Here is the beginning of the sense of ambivalence, and the potential for psychological maturity. The infant begins to realize that good and bad exist both within himself and within others. He also begins to trust that relationships can contain and manage conflict and difference without destroying friendship or love. With this growing awareness of the object, usually mother, as an important other person, the infant tries to internalize her as a defence against his fear of losing her. The nature of object relating at this time is therefore that of introjection. In Winnicott's terms, the infant begins to develop "a capacity for concern" (Winnicott, 1963a).

The working-through of this depressive position is never fully achieved, and at times of stress, disruption, trauma, or loss there can be a regression to the earlier paranoid–schizoid position, with its more primitive defences of splitting, projection, and blame. The ideal state of emotional maturity, therefore, is never actually reached, but the quest for integration and maturation continues throughout life.

The couple relationship

The committed couple relationship, because of its intensity, intimacy, and longevity, makes possible an interaction between two people at greater depth than any other, except for that of early infancy. It offers the opportunity for intensive attachment, which may allow each partner to be in touch again, usually unconsciously, with some of the experiences, good and bad, of early infancy. It also offers the unique combination of the opportunity to regress within the intimacy of the on-going sexual relationship and, at the same time, the opportunity for the responsibility of parenthood.

When a couple choose to make a committed relationship, there may be an unconscious recognition by each of them of disowned, denied, or projected parts of the self in the other. The unconscious choice of partner is made partly on the basis of the partner being a good receptacle for projective identification. This, of course, will be a shared or collusive choice, so that to some degree each spouse may carry and contain split-off and disowned aspects of the other. By making such a choice, by creating a marital fit, the couple may be said to be making an *unconscious contract* for the purposes of development *and* defence. Developmentally, the attraction for each is towards being in touch with or knowing more about repudiated aspects of the self as located in the other, and in doing so becoming more integrated. Defensively, the attraction for each may be an unconsciously shared collusion to retain certain splits and projections in a shared defence against shared anxieties.

This process, by which disowned aspects of the self are seen in the partner, is that of projective identification and is at work in all human relationships and in all couple relationships. The unconscious wisdom of locating projected parts of the self in the partner is that the potential exists to tangle with this attribute in the other, with a hope of eventually reintegrating that which had been projected.

Let me give a brief and simple illustration to show a predominantly developmental unconscious contract between a couple.

> Mr and Mrs Brown came for couple psychotherapy because of a shared and growing sense of dissatisfaction and disappointment in their relationship. Their initial attraction had been that of being opposites: he was passive, slow, and a painstaking planner; she was extrovert, active, and often quite chaotic. His career required him to be patient and careful, and to think in terms of months and years into the future; her career demanded quick thinking and fast decision-making. Initially both had been attracted by these differences, and they married with high expectations of their relationship. Slowly, however, dissatisfaction set in, and the very

differences that had initially attracted each to the other were now becoming the major source of disagreement and tension. Mrs Brown began to feel angry and restricted by her husband's slow pace and insistence on always making careful plans. Equally, Mr Brown was becoming increasingly resentful of his wife's extroversion and active life-style.

What emerged in the clinical work with this couple was that each partner attacked in the other that which was most feared but also most longed for. The husband feared his more asser-tive and active parts and had projected these attributes into his wife, who was an easy recipient of these qualities. Uncon-sciously, he had hoped that in the course of his relationship with her he could learn to be more at ease with these aspects of himself and reintegrate them. Mrs Brown feared the more re-flective, passive parts of herself, but she, too, had married with an unconscious hope of living with these aspects of herself in her husband and being enabled to take them back into herself. It is not difficult to see how useful Bion's concept of con-tainer/contained (Bion, 1962b, 1967) is in understanding the ordinary unconscious expectation and function of intimate re-lationships. However, the developmental aspect of the uncon-scious contract that had attracted this couple to each other had not been fulfilled, and unconsciously it was this failure that was the basis of their shared disappointment and frustra-tion. They needed the containment offered by the psychothera-pists in the course of couple psychotherapy to begin to take back their previously repudiated or projected parts. We began to feel that the psychotherapy was having a real impact on them when we heard about the changes in their sexual rela-tionship. Throughout their marriage, Mrs Brown had always been the more sexually active and interested partner, her hus-band the more passive, rarely, if ever, initiating sex. As the therapy progressed, we heard that this pattern between them was changing and that they could now both more easily take either the more passive or the more active roles, with the initial moves towards sex coming as often from Mr Brown as from his wife.

Outlined here, very simply, is the developmental potential of a good-enough couple relationship, with the more defensive aspects flexible enough to allow for a therapeutic intervention. Both partners, at the end of the psychotherapy, had a more comfortable relationship with their internal objects, and therefore their need to project parts of their inner world was reduced. This would, then, of course, influence the nature of their real external relationships. In this way, a couple relationship offers the potential of being, "the cradle for psychic development" (Lyons, chapter ten, this volume).

Defensive partner choice

Couple psychotherapists, however, are more likely to see relationships that are much more defensive and closed, unconsciously used by both partners to ward off unconscious anxieties. Such partnerships are anti-developmental and can be identified by the preponderance of the more primitive defences such as splitting, projection, blame, denial, idealization, and denigration.

Some may be so restricted as to feel almost as if the couple are fused. Neither partner is able to display any individuality or autonomy without the other feeling deeply threatened and rejected. The unconscious agreement in such a marital fit could be that the world outside is dangerous and hostile and that the only safe place is within the couple's relationship. One could say that both partners are made deeply anxious by, and therefore have to defend against, difference and separateness, which is then mutually projected outside the couple relationship, creating an external world then seen as dangerous and threatening.

Alternatively, relationships are seen where both partners constantly express only anger and hatred to each other. Often one or both have had a previous relationship that sounds as if it were very similar to the current one. The constant fights, abuse, hatred, and conflicts recounted and often actually displayed in the consulting room make it very difficult to understand why such a couple stay together. The partners in such a relationship may be said to be defending against commitment and intimacy. Good experiences can only be had outside the relationship, where they are felt to be more manageable because they can be made short-term and less committed.

And, lastly, relationships may be seen where the split is maintained between the couple. One partner will constantly express the need for independence, *unconsciously knowing* that the other will express the need for togetherness. In such a relationship, if the partner who was expressing the need for separateness began to seek an increase of intimacy from the other, the other would withdraw and demand more independence. *Between them* the couple maintain a system that enables them *both* to avoid whatever it is that they both fear.

Let me give an illustration.

Mr and Mrs Avon had been together for six years when they came for couple psychotherapy. The presenting problem was that their sexual relationship had all but ceased about a year earlier. The overt picture was of a husband who expressed a desire for sex and intimacy, and of a wife who constantly refused him. A few months into the therapy, Mrs Avon reported that a few evenings earlier they had gone out to dinner, had had a good evening, including a couple of bottles of wine, and on returning home she had seduced her husband. They had had exciting and mutually satisfying sexual intercourse. Mrs Avon went on to say that she was now feeling very confused and angry, because since that evening her husband had made no sexual approaches to her and had deflected her approaches towards him. Mr Avon was looking rather shocked and in a panic. He turned to his wife and said rather plaintively that he was very busy at work with a very demanding and important project and just had no energy left at the end of the day.

This reversal was extraordinary to observe and showed clearly, both to the couple and to the therapists, that the marital couple had unconsciously developed a collusive system that enabled them *both* to avoid whatever it was that sexual intimacy meant for them. As long as Mrs Avon refused his sexual advances, Mr Avon freely made them, knowing that he would be refused. Mrs Avon unconsciously knew that once she started to make sexual advances to her husband, he could be depended on to withdraw his sexual interest from her. *Between them* they ensured that sexual intimacy was avoided, with the overtly defensive behaviour only needing to be enacted by one of them on behalf of both.

I have described three types of marital fit: the fused marriage, the feuding marriage, and the split marriage. (This scheme follows that of Mattinson & Sinclair, 1979.) No single couple relationship could be delineated by simply using one of the three models suggested: real life is more interesting than that. Most relationships will have elements of all three, with perhaps a greater tendency towards one rather than either of the other two. In all three types, the predominant behaviour can be seen as a jointly collusive system maintained unconsciously by both partners to ward off an unspoken but shared anxiety or fear.

This concept of a *shared defence*, used by both partners to ward off a *shared fear or phantasy*, is central to the theory and practice of psychoanalytic couple psychotherapy.

Another way of making this point is to say that the couple between them develop a required (defensive) relationship in preference to an avoided but wished-for relationship that is feared because it is felt that it would result in a calamity. (This model was first used by Ezriel, 1956, to illustrate the nature of the psychoanalytic transference relationship.) What could be meant by the feared calamity? Let me return to Mr and Mrs Avon to illustrate it.

> The first clue came when Mr and Mrs Avon mentioned, in passing, that before sex had ceased they had briefly discussed the possibility of starting a family. They were both in their late twenties, so there seemed no immediate urgency about this issue, they said, but we were alerted. We learned over the course of the therapy that Mrs Avon was the second-oldest child of her family, and that her father had left her mother just a few months after she, Mrs Avon, was born. His regular visits to her mother were a constant reminder to Mrs Avon of whom she had lost, as well as a constant reminder that before her birth, her mother and father had maintained their relationship. We further learned that her mother had subsequently established a relationship with another man, who came to live in the family home and treated Mrs Avon very much as his own loved daughter. Suddenly this man left, established another relationship, and quickly had a child by his new partner.

From Mr Avon, we learned that for the first three years of his life he had been brought up by his mother and two indulgent aunts who lived with them. Father was away at the time working abroad. When father returned, Mr Avon and his parents moved into a new house, leaving behind the two aunts, and the parents quickly produced three more children to add to the family.

It emerged, therefore, that for both Mr and Mrs Avon the avoided relationship was that of a sexual relationship that resulted in the birth of a child. For both of them during early childhood the birth of a child had coincided with loss—in particular the loss of the attention of the parent of the opposite sex. Mrs Avon's father left just after her birth, and then her substitute father left and had a child by another woman. For Mr Avon, the birth of his siblings coincided with the loss of the sole attention of his mother, as well as the loss of his aunts and of his original home.

For this couple, then, the required relationship or shared defensive behaviour was that of a non-sexual relationship. The avoided relationship was that of procreative sexuality. And the shared phantasy or feared calamity was that if they were to produce a child, the other would leave them, either physically or emotionally. Paradoxically, it was as if, in phantasy, procreative sexuality was life-threatening rather than life-creating.

However, the choice of each other as partners—their unconscious contract—was based on unconsciously recognized mutual anxieties and conflicts. Both unconsciously recognized in the other a shared developmental task: to trust that they could engaged in procreative sexuality, produce a child, and *not* lose the love of the partner.

Clinical practice

Therapeutic understanding and change occurs in the crucible of the transference and countertransference relationship inherent in the patient–therapist encounter. Psychic change is brought about by the modification of the patient's internal world by interpreting the transference relationship, which is an expression of that internal world. This is no less true for the couple psychotherapist than for the individual psychoanalytic psychotherapist.

Following Klein's views on transference (Klein, 1952), Betty Joseph, in writing about individual psychoanalytic practice, reminds us that the understanding of the transference

> must include everything that the patients brings into the (therapeutic) relationship. What he brings in can best be gauged by our focusing our attention on what is going on within the relationship, how he is using the analyst, alongside and beyond what he is saying. Much of our understanding of the transference comes through our understanding of how our patients act on us to feel things for many varied reasons; how they try to draw us into their defensive systems; how they unconsciously act out with us in the transference, trying to get us to act out with them; how they convey aspects of their inner world built up from infancy—elaborated in childhood and adulthood, experiences often beyond the use of words. [Joseph, 1985]

Working with couples in conjoint psychotherapy offers a rich but extremely complex labyrinth of transference relationships. There will be the individual transferences towards the two therapists separately, and the marital transference, based on the shared phantasies and defences, towards the two therapists separately. But most important will be the individual and the marital transferences towards *the two therapists as a couple* (Ruszczynski, 1992).

Klein developed the notion of a child's internal world occupied by figures derived from early real experiences distorted by projections and introjections. These figures will, from very early on, include the parental couple—both real and in phantasy. This internal couple and the individual's relationship to it will influence the hopes, anxieties, and expectations that will play a part in the choice of partner in adulthood. It can be speculated that there will be some degree of overlap in this internal object relation between the two people who find themselves attracted to each other and who decide to establish a committed relationship. The individual and the shared internal couple images will be transferred onto the therapist couple in the course of couple psychotherapy. This transference and the subsequent countertransference will offer access to the inner worlds of the two partners and to the nature of their object relations and couple interaction.

Let me give an illustration.

During the course of psychotherapy with Mr and Mrs Jones, my female co-therapist, unfortunately and rather suddenly, had to tell them that due to unforeseeable circumstances she would be absent from the therapy for the following six weeks. She gave her apologies, and we waited for the couples' reaction, assuming that they would express some disappointment or even anger, or, at the very least, some curiosity in the reasons for her forthcoming absence. The couple were completely unmoved by the news and ignored it. When we eventually found an opportunity to comment on this total lack of reaction, they said that the news of my co-therapist's impending absence was irrelevant, because I would go on seeing them. It was as if they could not see us as two separate people to whom they could react in different ways. They seemed, in effect, to deny my colleague's forthcoming absence and see only my continued presence. After the session my co-therapist and I wondered whether the couple had serious difficulties with difference and separateness, fearing that these might lead to anxieties about rejection and abandonment, and that their shared defence was a very powerful splitting and denial.

During my colleague's absence, I commented on her empty chair as often as the material allowed, and in that sense kept her alive, at least for myself. Slowly, I realized that in their material the couple were beginning to tell me how difficult they found it to feel and express any differences between them. For example, Mrs Jones said that she had recently been unable to allow herself to mourn the death of a close relative, because Mr Jones had not known this aunt and therefore would have no particular feelings about her loss. Mr Jones reported that he had been unable to share with his wife his increasing frustration and unhappiness about his work, because he knew how happy and settled she was in her career.

The internal object relation shared by our patients appeared to be a couple who had to violently split off and expel any difference or disagreement, because autonomy or differentiation was feared as a threat to the relationship. Furthermore, the only way they could express their negative feelings about the loss of one of their therapists and how this would possibly frustrate the work of the psychotherapy was unconsciously through their material in the sessions. Mr and Mrs Jones had originally presented themselves for couple psychotherapy because they had almost no sex life, and Mrs Jones' age was forcing her to think about the possibility of starting a family, but they could not even discuss this issue. Their shared internal image was of a sterile couple who were not even sexually different enough to entertain the possibility of creative intercourse, sexual or otherwise. The active differentation, then, between myself and my co-therapist, highlighted by her impending individual absence, had to be dealt with by splitting and denial. Equally split off and denied was any feelings they had about the disruption to the therapy caused by her absence.

Countertransference and projective identification

Hand in hand with transference is, of course, countertransference. The term here is used in its more contemporary sense as referring to the understanding that some of the feelings aroused in the psychotherapist are unconsciously projected into him by the patient. The unconscious hope is that the container/therapist can manage and process projected feelings, which can then be introjected by the patient, along with the possibility that he (the patient) may be able to do likewise. As Freud wrote, without ever going on to develop the thought, "everyone possesses in his own unconscious an instrument with which he can interpret the utterances of the unconscious in other people" (Freud, 1913i).

The concept of countertransference is closely related to that of projective identification, which originated in the work of

Klein (1946). She used the term to describe a primitive mechanism of defence. Bion developed the concept by showing that in addition to being a defence mechanism, projective identification was also the first mode of communication between mother and infant. This understanding is now widely used in clinical practice, and I will quote Ogden, who usefully defines the concept of projective identification in its full breadth:

> Projective identification is a psychological process that is at once a type of defence, a model of communication, a primitive form of object relation and a pathway for psychological change. As a defence, projective identification serves to create a psychological distance from unwanted, often frightening aspects of the self. As a mode of communication, projective identification is a process by which feelings congruent with one's own are induced in another person, thereby creating a sense of being understood, or "at one with" the other person. As a type of object relations, projective identification constitutes a way of being with and relating to a partially separate object. Finally, as a pathway for psychological change, projective identification is a process by which feelings like those that one is struggling with are psychologically processed by another person and made available for reinternalisation in an altered form. [Ogden, 1982]

At the Tavistock Institute of Marital Studies, there has developed a particular way in which the couple psychotherapist's countertransference feelings, evoked by the patient's projective identification, can be used in couple psychotherapy (Mattinson, 1975). This starts from a principle originally put forward by Harold Searles (1955), who wrote: "The processes at work currently in the relationship between patient and therapist are often reflected in the relationship between therapist and supervisor . . . I shall refer to this phenomenon as the reflection process."

At the TIMS, this has been adapted for use in psychotherapy with couples. If the therapist couple can be open and honest in their discussion about their work with any particular couple, including a discussion of the feelings aroused between them as co-therapists, then they may reflect the interaction of the marital couple in their own therapist relationship: "facets of

the interaction between the married pair . . . 'get into' the interaction between the [therapists]" (Mattinson, 1975).

If the therapist couple can contain (rather than act out),
reflect on, and process that which has been projected into them,
they may subsequently be able to help the patient couple do
likewise, either through verbal interpretation of that which is
now better understood or through non-interpretive interventions and management of the therapy. Either way, the therapists can convey a containment, processing, and understanding
of that which has unconsciously been projected into them, and
so the patient couple can introject in a modified form feelings
that had previously carried so much anxiety that they had to
be projected. The couple will also introject the beginning of the
capacity to manage better their own containment and processing of frightening feelings.

Let me give two illustrations.

Mr and Mrs Smith came to psychotherapy saying that
their problem was the near-impossibility of their finding
time in their very busy schedules to be together, either as
a couple or as parents to their two young children. Both
led busy and demanding professional and social lives and
had no time left for each other. This dynamic inevitably
became enacted in the therapeutic process, whereby one
or other of them would have pressing appointments
elsewhere, which prevented them attending some sessions.

As the therapy progressed, my co-therapist and I realized
that we were spending less and less time between sessions
talking together about our work with this couple—a
practice we view as essential to joint couple
psychotherapy. We would arrange to meet, and one of us
would forget. Or we would meet, and then find that one or
the other of us had only a few minutes because of
something else that had to be attended to. It did not take
much to realize that in the countertransference we were
caught up in reflecting the couple's problem, projected
into our co-therapist relationship. We could not be clear as
to why this was the required (defensive) relationship, but
we resolved to meet regularly and spend a reasonable
amount of time discussing our work with this couple—our

usual practice. Within a few weeks we began to hear from the couple that they were both dropping some of their outside activities so as to have more time together as a couple and as parents. Not a single session of therapy was ever missed again.

Given that we did not understand the anxiety that underlay the defensive non-meeting relationship, it is difficult to explain fully how this change came about. However, once my co-therapist and I became conscious of what we were unconsciously acting out as a reflection of the couple and then managed to regularly find time together, we must have communicated our increased togetherness to our patients through the subsequent nature of our interaction together as a therapist pair in the consulting room with them. In the same way that we had initially unconsciously identified with the couple's problem projected into us, so the couple were able to unconsciously identify and introject our management of it.

This example illustrates that the management of a therapy can in itself produce therapeutic benefits.

A further example may show more clearly the reflection process, based on countertransference, and its use in couple psychotherapy.

My female co-therapist and I had been seeing a couple for about four months. They were in their early forties, had four children in their early teens, and had been referred to the TIMS for couple psychotherapy by a family therapist, whom they had consulted because of their growing worry about one of their daughters who was stealing from within the home.

Mr and Mrs Adams were a rather dour, depressed, almost frozen couple, who found it very difficult to talk with each other. They tended to give very brief statements in monologue, and neither was able to add or respond to what the other said. The sessions were often very stilted and slow, and we as therapists would often find ourselves caught up in the very tense and anxious atmosphere that pervaded the consulting room. We had noted, in our private discussions about this couple, the very fragmented and incoherent nature of their interaction, but we had not really understood it. We *did* know that Mrs Adams had had a number of depressive episodes, some of which had been psychotic in nature and had resulted in hospitalization.

During one session I found myself particularly uncomfortable. I began to feel frozen, but full of thoughts and feelings that I felt I could not make use of. I know that this is unusual for me: I usually feel freer to engage in a session. As I reflected on what I was experiencing, I suddenly realized that I was remaining silent because I was frightened that if I were to say what I was thinking and feeling, my co-therapist would not like what I had said, and that we would end up disagreeing and even fighting!

I work with this particular co-therapist colleague regularly and know that such a possibility was highly unlikely. My fears were anomalous, and I began to wonder whether they were a reflection of the couple's unspoken fears. This self-reflection suddenly seemed to free me: I offered an interpretation, wondering with the couple whether they were very frightened to engage in a dialogue with each other because they feared how the other would receive and react to what they said. Initially there was a silence, but then Mrs Adams said that she had always felt very frightened to tell her husband when she was angered or irritated by him. She feared that he would dismiss her comments as being groundless, saying that she only felt this way because of her depressive illness. In this way, she said, it was almost as if he were "robbing her" of the way that she was feeling. (Note that the original presenting problem, which had taken this family to a therapist, was the stealing within the home by one of their children.) Mr Adams looked at his wife and nodded. In previous sessions the couple had demonstrated how Mrs Adams' complaints about her husband would often, indeed, be relegated by her husband as simply to do with her psychiatric illness. Mr Adams then said that he found it very difficult to think of his wife's depression as anything other than an illness. What frightened him about it, he said, was that if he were to talk about it he might discover that he was feeling very similar to the way in which she was feeling, and sometimes perhaps even worse than she was feeling.

This couple could be said to share an internal image of a coupling that was frozen and stilted, with a prevalent fear that any form of communication would be dangerous, violent, and possibly destructive. Any form of interaction, therefore, had to be very restrained and limited. Unconsciously projecting this, the couple had evoked in me the frozen silent state that only on reflection could I process and understand and then make available to them in a form that included a recognition of the anxiety underlying it. Recognizing this was the first step to beginning to understand the nature of their relationship.

IN SUMMARY

A couple who choose to make a committed relationship are likely to share an unconscious phantasy or image of the nature of "marriage"—not necessarily of external world marriage, but of the nature of linking, connecting, and relating. In part, it will be this shared unconscious image of the internal couple that will bring the partners together and structure their attachment to each other. The nature of the internal object relations will then substantially influence the nature of the couple's marital relationship.

In the course of couple psychotherapy the patient couple will project onto the therapist couple images and phantasies stemming from these shared internalized object relations. Marital transference interpretations (Ruszczynski, 1992) will promote a modification of the internal images of "marriage" and so free the real world relationship from unconscious fears and phantasies. The couple relationship will then be freer to perform the ordinarily therapeutic containment of human relating.

REFERENCES

Adelman, J. (1985). This is and is not Cressida: The characterisation of Cressida. In: S. N. Garner, C. Kahane, & M. Sprengnether (Eds.), *The (M)other Tongue: Essays in Feminist Psychological Interpretation* (pp. 119–141). Ithaca, NY: Cornell University Press.

Allenby, A. I. (1961). The Church and the analyst. *Journal of Analytical Psychology*, 6: 137–156.

Allingham, M. (1987). *Unconscious Contracts: A Psychoanalytical Theory of Society*. London: Routledge and Kegan Paul.

Astbury, B. E. (1955). Foreword. In: K. Bannister, A. Lyons, L. Pincus, J. Robb, A. Shooter, & J. Stephens, *Social Casework in Marital Problems*. London: Tavistock Publications.

Attwood, M. (1989). *Cat's Eye*. London: Virago Press.

Bannister, K., Lyons, A., Pincus, L., Robb, J., Shooter, A., & Stephens, J. (1955). *Social Casework in Marital Problems*. London: Tavistock Publications.

Bannister, K., & Pincus, L. (1965). *Shared Phantasy in Marital Problems*. London: Institute of Marital Studies.

Bateson, G. (1973). *Steps to an Ecology of Mind*. London: Paladin.

Bion, W. (1952). Group dynamics: A review. *International Journal of Psycho-Analysis*, 33: 235–247.

_____ (1955). Language and the schizophrenic. In: M. Klein, P. Heimann, & R. Money-Kyrle (Eds.), *New Directions in Psycho-Analysis* (pp. 220–259). London: Tavistock Publications. [Reprinted London: Karnac Books, 1989.]

_____ (1961). *Experiences in Groups*. London: Tavistock Publications.

_____ (1962a). *Learning from Experience*. London: Heinemann. [Reprinted London: Karnac Books, 1984.]

_____ (1962b). A theory of thinking. *International Journal of Psycho-Analysis*, 43: 306–310. [Reprinted in: *Second Thoughts* (pp. 110–119). London: Karnac Books, 1984.]

_____ (1967). *Second Thoughts: Selected Papers on Psycho-Analysis*. London: Heinemann. [Reprinted London: Karnac Books, 1984.]

_____ (1970). *Attention and Interpretation*. London: Tavistock Publications. [Reprinted London: Karnac Books, 1984.]

_____ (1978). *Four Discussions with W. R. Bion.* Scotland: Clunie Press.

Blos, P. (1985). *Son and Father: Before and Beyond the Oedipus Complex.* New York: Free Press.

Bott, E. (1957). Acknowledgments. In: *Family and Social Network* (pp. ix–xi). London: Tavistock Publications.

Bowlby, J. (1969). *Attachment and Loss. Vol. 1. Attachment.* London: Hogarth Press.

_____ (1973a). *Attachment and Loss. Vol. 2. Separation: Anxiety and Anger.* London: Hogarth Press.

_____ (1973b). Self reliance and some conditions that promote it. In: R. Gosling (Ed.), *Support, Innovation and Autonomy: Tavistock Clinic Golden Jubilee Papers* (pp. 23–48). London: Tavistock Publications.

_____ (1980). *Attachment and Loss. Vol. 3. Loss: Sadness and Repression.* London: Hogarth Press.

Britton, R. (1989). The missing link: Parental sexuality in the Oedipus complex. In: R. Britton, M. Feldman, & E. O'Shaughnessy, *The Oedipus Complex Today: Clinical Implications,* edited by J. Steiner (pp. 83–101). London: Karnac Books.

Carpy, D. (1989). Tolerating the countertransference: A mutative process. *International Journal of Psycho-Analysis, 70*: 287–294.

Clulow, C. F. (1982). *To Have and to Hold.* Aberdeen: Aberdeen University Press.

_____ (1985). *Marital Therapy: An Inside View.* Aberdeen: Aberdeen University Press.

_____ (Ed.) (1990). *Marriage: Disillusion and Hope.* London: Karnac Books.

Clulow, C. F., Dearnley, B., & Balfour, F. (1986). Shared phantasy and therapeutic structure in a brief marital psychotherapy. *British Journal of Psychotherapy, 3*: 124–132.

Clulow, C. F., & Mattinson, J. (1989). *Marriage Inside Out.* Harmondsworth, Middlexex: Penguin.

Clulow, C. F., & Vincent, C. M. (1987). *In the Child's Best Interests.* London: Tavistock, Sweet and Maxwell.

Colman, W. (1989). *On Call.* Aberdeen: Aberdeen University Press.

Daniell, D. (1985). Love and work: Complementary aspects of personal identity. *International Journal of Social Economics, 12*: 48–55.

Dicks, H. (1967). *Marital Tensions.* London: Routledge and Kegan Paul.

_____ (1970). *Fifty Years of the Tavistock Clinic.* London: Routledge and Kegan Paul.

Ezriel, H. (1956). Experimentation within the psycho-analytic session. *British Journal for the Philosophy of Science, 7:* 29–48.

Feldman, M. (1989). The Oedipus complex: Manifestations in the inner world and the therapeutic situation. In: R. Britton, M. Feldman, & E. O'Shaughnessy, *The Oedipus Complex Today: Clinical Implications,* edited by J. Steiner (pp. 103–128). London: Karnac Books.

Flügel, J. C. (1921). *The Psychoanalytic Study of the Family.* London: Hogarth Press.

Fordham, M. (1978). *Jungian Psychotherapy: A Study in Analytical Psychology.* Chichester: John Wiley. [Reprinted London: Karnac Books, 1986.]

Forster, E. M. (1924). *A Passage to India.* Harmondsworth, Middlesex: Penguin.

Freud, S. (1895d) (with Breuer, J.). *Studies on Hysteria.* In: *Standard Edition of the Complete Psychological Works of Sigmund Freud, Vol. 2.* London: Hogarth Press, 1950–1974.

_____ (1900a). *The Interpretation of Dreams.* In: *S.E.,* Vols. 4–5 (pp. 1–627).

_____ (1909b). Analysis of a phobia in a five-year-old boy. In: *S.E.,* Vol. *10* (pp. 1–149).

_____ (1913c). On beginning the treatment (Further recommendations on the technique of psycho-analysis, 1). In: *S.E., Vol. 12* (pp. 121–144).

_____ (1913i). The disposition to obsessional neurosis. In: *S.E., Vol. 12* (pp. 311–326).

_____ (1915e). The unconscious. In: *S.E., Vol. 14* (pp. 159–215).

_____ (1917e). Mourning and melancholia. In: *S.E., Vol. 14* (pp. 237–260).

_____ (1916–17). *Introductory Lectures on Psycho-Analysis:* Lecture XXVIII: Analytic Therapy. In: *S.E., Vol. 16* (pp. 448–463).

_____ (1921c). *Group Psychology and the Analysis of the Ego.* In: *S.E., Vol. 18* (pp. 65–143).

_____ (1923b). *The Ego and the Id.* In: *S.E., Vol. 19* (pp. 1–66).

_____ (1923e). The infantile genital organization. In: *S.E., Vol. 19* (pp. 141–145).

_____ (1924d). The dissolution of the Oedipus complex. In: *S.E., Vol. 19* (pp. 173–179).

_____ (1925j). Some psychical consequences of the anatomical distinction between the sexes. In: *S.E., Vol. 19* (pp. 241–258).

_____ (1926d [1925]). *Inhibitions, Symptoms and Anxiety.* In: *S.E., Vol. 20* (pp. 75–175).

_____ (1931b). Female sexuality. In: *S.E., Vol. 21* (pp. 221–243).

_____ (1933a). *New Introductory Lectures on Psycho-Analysis.* In: *S.E., Vol. 22* (pp. 1–182).

_____ (1940a [1938]). An outline of psychoanalysis. In: *S.E., Vol. 23* (pp. 141–207).

Gay, P. (1988). *Freud: A Life for Our Time.* London: J. M. Dent.

Giovacchini, P. (1961). Resistance and external object relations. *International Journal of Psycho-Analysis, 42*: 246–254.

Greenberg, J. R., & Mitchell, S. A. (1983). *Object Relations in Psychoanalytic Theory.* Cambridge, MA: Harvard University Press.

Guthrie, L., & Mattinson, J. (1971). *Brief Casework with a Marital Problem.* London: Institute of Marital Studies.

Haldane, D. (1991). Holding hope in trust: A review of the publications of the Tavistock Institute of Marital Studies, 1955–1991. *Journal of Social Work Practice, 5:* 199–204.

Hartman, H. (1958). *Ego Psychology and the Problems of Adaptation.* New York: International Universities Press.

Heimann, P. (1950). On countertransference. *International Journal of Psycho-Analysis, 31:* 81–84.

Hillman, J. (1964). Betrayal. In: *Loose Ends* (pp. 63–81). Dallas: Spring (1975).

Howell, D. (1979). Individuation and the shadow. Unpublished Lecture given at the Analytical Society Club.

Institute of Marital Studies (1962). *The Marital Relationship as a Focus for Casework.* London: IMS.

Jacobi, J. (1942). *The Psychology of C. G. Jung.* London: Routledge and Kegan Paul.

Jacques, E. (1955). Social systems as a defence against persecutory and depressive anxiety. In: M. Klein, P. Heimann, & R. Money-Kyrle (Eds.), *New Directions in Psycho-Analysis* (pp. 478–498). London: Tavistock Publications. [Reprinted London: Karnac Books, 1989.]

James, C. (1984). Bion's "containing" and Winnicott's "holding" in the context of the group matrix. *International Journal of Group Psychotherapy, 34:* 201–213.

Joseph, B. (1985). Transference: The total situation. *International Journal of Psycho-Analysis, 66:* 447–454. [Reprinted in: E. Bott Spillius & M. Feldman (Eds.), *Psychic Equilibrium and Psychic Change: Selected Papers of Betty Joseph* (pp. 156–167). London: Tavistock/Routledge, 1989.]

_____ (1988). Object relations in clinical practice. In: E. Bott Spillius & M. Feldman (Eds.), *Psychic Equilibrium and Psychic Change: Selected Papers of Betty Joseph* (pp. 156–167). London: Tavistock/Routledge, 1989.

_____ (1989). *Psychic Equilibrium and Psychic Change: Selected Papers of Betty Joseph*, edited by E. Bott Spillius & M. Feldman. London: Tavistock/ Routledge.

Jung, C. G. (1954–1990). *The Collected Works of C. G. Jung*. London: Routledge and Kegan Paul.

_____ (1917). The psychology of the unconscious. *C.W.*, *Vol. 7* (pp. 3–117).

_____ (1921). Psychological types. *C.W.*, *Vol. 6*.

_____ (1925). Marriage as a psychological relationship. *C.W.*, *Vol. 17* (pp. 187–201).

_____ (1929). The relation between the ego and the unconscious. *C.W.*, *Vol. 7* (pp. 121–239).

_____ (1934a). Individuation. *C.W.*, *Vol. 7* (pp. 171–239).

_____ (1934b). The development of the personality. *C.W.*, *Vol. 17* (pp. 167–186).

_____ (1939). Conscious, unconscious, and individuation. *C.W.*, *Vol. 9, Part 1* (pp. 273–289).

_____ (1940). The psychology of the child archetype. *C.W.*, *Vol. 9* (pp. 151–181).

_____ (1944). Psychology and alchemy. *C.W.*, *Vol. 12*

_____ (1946). Psychology of the transference. *C.W.*, *Vol. 16* (pp. 163–323).

_____ (1958). The transcendent function. *C.W.*, *Vol. 8* (pp. 67–91).

Klein, M. (1945). The Oedipus complex in the light of early anxieties. *International Journal of Psycho-Analysis, 26*: pp. 11–33. [Reprinted in: *The Writings of Melanie Klein, Vol. 1*. London: Hogarth Press, 1975; reprinted London: Karnac Books, 1992.]

_____ (1946). Notes on some schizoid mechanisms. *International Journal of Psycho-Analysis, 27*: 99–110. [Reprinted in: *The Writings of Melanie Klein, Vol. 3*. London: Hogarth Press, 1975.]

_____ (1952). The origins of transference. *International Journal of Psycho-Analysis, 33*: 433–438. [Reprinted in: *The Writings of Melanie Klein, Vol. 3*. London: Hogarth Press, 1975.]

Kohon, G. (1986). Prefatory remarks. In: G. Kohon (Ed.), *The British School of Psychoanalysis: The Independent Tradition* (pp. 19–23). London: Free Association Books.

Lampl-de-Groot, J. (1927). The evolution of the Oedipus complex in women. *International Journal of Psycho-Analysis, 9* (1928): 332–345.

Laplanche, J., & Pontalis, J. B. (1973). *The Language of Psycho-analysis.* London: Hogarth Press. [Reprinted London: Karnac Books, 1988.]

Lively, P. (1977). *The Road to Lichfield.* Harmondsworth, Middlesex: Penguin.

Main, T. F. (1966). Mutual projection in a marriage. *Comprehensive Psychiatry, 7* (5), 432–449.

Mainprice, J. (1974). *Marital Interaction and Some Illnesses in Children.* London: Institute of Marital Studies.

Mattinson, J. (1970). *Marriage and Mental Handicap.* London: Duckworth/Institute of Marital Studies (1975).

———— (1975). *The Reflection Process in Casework Supervision.* London: Institute of Marital Studies. [Republished 1992.]

———— (1988). *Work, Love and Marriage: The Impact of Unemployment.* London: Duckworth.

Mattinson, J., & Sinclair, I. (1979). *Mate and Stalemate.* Oxford: Blackwell [London: Institute of Marital Studies, 1981].

McGuire, W., & Hull, R. F. C. (Eds.) (1978). *C. G. Jung Speaking: Interviews and Encounters.* London: Thames and Hudson.

Meltzer, D. (1966). The relation of anal masturbation to projective identification *International Journal of Psycho-Analysis, 47,* 335–342.

Meltzer, D. (1967). *The Psycho-Analytical Process.* London: Heinemann.

———— (1978). Freud's clinical development. In: *The Kleinian Development, Part I.* Perthshire: Clunie Press.

———— (1982). The conceptual distinction between projective identification (Klein) and container/contained (Bion). *Journal of Child Psychotherapy, 8:* 185–202.

———— (1988). Unpublished talk given to the Society of Analytical Psychology.

Menzies, I. E. P. (1949). Factors affecting family breakdown in urban communities. *Human Relations, 11* (4): 363–374. [Reprinted in: I. Menzies Lyth, *Containing Anxiety in Institutions: Selected Essays.* London: Free Association Books, 1989.]

———— (1970). *The Functioning of Social Systems as a Defence against Anxiety.* London: Tavistock Institute of Human Relations.

Miller, A. (1983). *The Drama of the Gifted Child and the Search for the True Self.* London: Faber and Faber.

Milner, M. (1955). The role of illusion in symbol formation. In: M. Klein, P. Heimann, & R. Money-Kyrle (Eds.), *New Directions in Psycho-Analysis* (pp. 82–108). London: Tavistock Publications [reprinted London: Karnac Books, 1989]. [Also reprinted in: M. Milner, *The Suppressed Madness of Sane Men* (pp. 83–113). London: Tavistock Publications, 1987.]

Minuchin, S. (1984). A day in court. *The Family Networker, 8* (6): 32–41.

Moggach, D. (1983). *Porky.* Harmondsworth, Middlesex: Penguin.

Morgan, M. E. (1992). Therapist gender and psychoanalytic couple psychotherapy. *Sexual and Marital Therapy, 7* (2): 141–156.

Nicholson, N. (1973). *Portrait of a Marriage.* London: Weidenfeld and Nicholson.

Obholzer, A. (1987). Institutional dynamics and resistance to change. *Psychoanalytic Psychotherapy, 2*: 201–206.

Ogden, T. (1982). *Projective Identification and Psychotherapeutic Technique.* New York: Jason Aronson.

O'Shaughnessy, E. (1989). The invisible Oedipus complex. In: R. Britton, M. Feldman, & E. O'Shaughnessy, *The Oedipus Complex Today: Clinical Implications,* edited by J. Steiner (pp. 129–150). London: Karnac Books.

Pincus, L. (Ed.) (1960). *Marriage: Studies in Emotional Conflict and Growth.* London: Methuen/Institute of Marital Studies, 1973.

Ruszczynski, S. (1991). Unemployment and marriage: The psychological meaning of work. *Journal of Social Work Practice, 5*: 19–30.

_____ (1992). Some notes towards a psychoanalytic understanding of the couple relationship. *Psychoanalytic Psychotherapy, 6* (1): 33–48.

Samuels, A. (1985). *Jung and the Post-Jungians.* London: Routledge and Kegan Paul.

Sandler, J., & Sandler, A.-M. (1978). On the development of object relationships and affects. *International Journal of Psycho-Analysis, 59*: 285–296.

Searles, H. (1955). The informational value of the supervisor's emotional experience. In: *Collected Papers on Schizophrenia and Related Subjects* (pp. 157–176). London: Hogarth Press, 1965. [Reprinted London: Karnac Books, 1986.]

Segal, H. (1989). Introduction. In: R. Britton, M. Feldman, & E. O'Shaughnessy, *The Oedipus Complex Today: Clinical Implications,* edited by J. Steiner (pp. 1–10). London: Karnac Books.

Shuttleworth, J. (1989). Psychoanalytic theory and infant development. In: L. Miller, M. Rustin, M. Rustin, & J. Shuttleworth (Eds.), *Closely Observed Infants* (pp. 22–51). London: Duckworth.

Simon, B. (1991). Is the Oedipus complex still the corner-stone of psychoanalysis? Three obstacles to answering the question. *Journal of the American Psychoanalytic Association, 39*: 641–668.

Skynner, R. (1969). Indications for and against conjoint family therapy. *International Journal of Social Psychiatry, 15*: 245–249.

Steiner, J. (Ed.) (1989). *The Oedipus Complex Today: Clinical Implications*, by R. Britton, M. Feldman, & E. O'Shaughnessy. London: Karnac Books.

Sutherland, J. D. (1963). Object relations theory and the conceptual model of psychoanalysis. *British Journal of Medical Psychology, 36*: 109–124.

Symington, N. (1986). *The Analytic Experience*. London: Free Association Books.

Williams, M. (1989). The archetypes in marriage. In: A. Samuels (Ed.), *Psychopathology: Contemporary Jungian Perspectives* (pp. 291–307). London: Routledge and Kegan Paul.

Winnicott, D. (1947). Hate in the countertransference. *International Journal of Psycho-Analysis, 30*: 69–74. [Reprinted in: *Through Paediatrics to Psycho-Analysis: Collected Papers*. London: Hogarth Press, 1958; republished 1975. Reprinted London: Karnac Books, 1992.]

_____ (1958). *Through Paediatrics to Psycho-Analysis: Collected Papers*. London: Hogarth Press. [Republished 1975. Reprinted London: Karnac Books, 1992.]

_____ (1960a). The theory of the parent–infant relationship. *International Journal of Psycho-Analysis, 41*: 585–595. [Reprinted in: *The Maturational Process and the Facilitating Environment*. London: Hogarth Press, 1965. Reprinted London: Karnac Books, 1990.]

_____ (1960b). Ego distortions in terms of true and false self. In: *The Maturational Process and the Facilitating Environment*. London: Hogarth Press, 1965. [Reprinted London: Karnac Books, 1990.]

_____ (1963a). The development of the capacity for concern. In: *The Maturational Process and the Facilitating Environment*. London: Hogarth Press, 1965. [Reprinted London: Karnac Books, 1990.]

_____ (1963b). Psychotherapy of character disorders. In: *The Maturational Process and the Facilitating Environment*. London: Hogarth Press, 1965. [Reprinted London: Karnac Books, 1990.]

_____ (1965). *The Maturational Process and the Facilitating Environment*. London: Hogarth Press. [Reprinted London: Karnac Books, 1990.]

_____ (1967a). Mirror-role of mother and family in child development. In: *Playing and Reality*. London: Tavistock Publications, 1971. [Republished London: Penguin, 1974.]

_____ (1967b). The location of cultural experience. *International Journal of Psycho-Analysis*, *48*: 368–372. [Reprinted in: *Playing and Reality*. London: Tavistock Publications, 1971; republished London: Penguin, 1974.]

_____ (1968). Communication between infant and mother, and mother and infant, compared and contrasted. In: W. G. Joffe (Ed.), *What Is Psychoanalysis?* (pp. 15–25). London: Balliere, Tindall and Cassell.

_____ (1971). *Playing and Reality*. London: Tavistock Publications. [Republished London: Penguin, 1974.]

_____ (1974). Fear of breakdown. *International Review of Psycho-Analysis*, *1*: 103–107.

_____ (1975). Quoted by M. Masud R. Khan, in: Introduction to 1975 republication of D. Winnicott, *Through Paediatrics to Psycho-Analysis: Collected Papers* (pp. xi–xxxxviii). London: Hogarth Press, 1958. [Reprinted London: Karnac Books, 1992.]

Woodhouse, D. L. (1990). The Tavistock Institute of Marital Studies: Evolution of a marital agency. In: C. Clulow (Ed.), *Marriage: Disillusion and Hope* (pp. 69–119). London: Karnac Books, 1990.

Woodhouse, D. L., & Pengelly, P. J. C. (1991). *Anxiety and the Dynamics of Collaboration*. Aberdeen: Aberdeen University Press.

Zinkin, L. (1979). Individuation and Adolescence. Unpublished lecture given to Analytical Society Club.

Zinner, J., & Shapiro, R. (1972). Projective identification as a mode of perception and behaviour in families of adolescents. *International Journal of Psycho-Analysis*, *53*: 523–530.

INDEX

Printed in the United States
by Baker & Taylor Publisher Services

Printed in the United States
by Baker & Taylor Publisher Services